Basics of Hypoglycemia

Edited by Alok Raghav

Published in London, United Kingdom

Basics of Hypoglycemia
http://dx.doi.org/10.5772/intechopen.95724
Edited by Alok Raghav

Contributors
Daniel Arturo Martínez-Piña, Gustavo Alexis Alvarado-Fernández, Edith González-Guevara, Carlos Castillo-Pérez, Gerardo Romero-Luna, Jorge Alejandro Torres-Ríos, Yasin Simsek, Emre Urhan, Rimma Shaginian, James Richardson, Ala' Abu-Odeh, Dalal Alnatour, Leen Fino, Dennis R.A. Mans, Anujka Selea Zivojinovic

First published in London, United Kingdom, 2022 by IntechOpen
IntechOpen is the global imprint of INTECHOPEN LIMITED, registered in England and Wales, registration number: 11086078, 5 Princes Gate Court, London, SW7 2QJ, United Kingdom

British Library Cataloguing-in-Publication Data
A catalogue record for this book is available from the British Library

Additional hard and PDF copies can be obtained from orders@intechopen.com

Basics of Hypoglycemia
Edited by Alok Raghav
p. cm.
Print ISBN 978-1-80355-897-4
Online ISBN 978-1-80355-898-1
eBook (PDF) ISBN 978-1-80355-899-8

Meet the editor

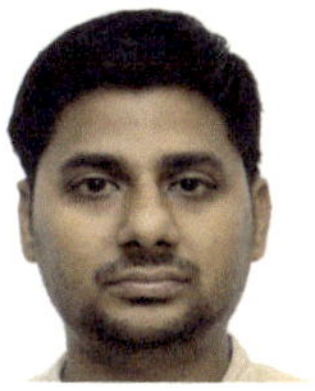

Dr. Alok Raghav obtained his doctoral degree in Endocrinology from Rajiv Gandhi Centre for Diabetes and Endocrinology, J.N. Medical College, Aligarh Muslim University (AMU), India. He worked as a project scientist at the Indian Institute of Technology in Kanpur, India. He has more than ten years of research experience in the field of glycobiology and diabetes mellitus. He is currently a Scientist C at the Multidisciplinary Research Unit (sponsored by the Department of Health Research, Ministry of Health and Family Welfare, New Delhi), GSVM Medical College Kanpur, India. He is also an associate editor and editor for several peer-reviewed journals, including *Frontiers in Endocrinology, Frontiers in Public Health,* and *PLOS One.*

Contents

Preface

Glucose is the crucial metabolic fuel that helps in maintaining brain homeostasis. Likewise, other organs of the body also require a continuous supply of arterial glucose for maintaining adequate functions. Potential comorbidities can arise due to interruption of this glucose supply, such as low blood sugar, known as hypoglycemia. Major causes of hypoglycemia include diabetes mellitus, non-islet cell tumors, alcohol, drugs, severe illness, and hormone deficiencies.

This book describes the fundamental concept of hypoglycemia and reflects the wide range of research currently being practiced in the field of diabetes mellitus. Although most of the concepts of hypoglycemia are applicable to diabetes mellitus and other comorbidities, we hope that this book will appeal to a broad spectrum of readers. It begins with an overview of hypoglycemia, which is the most important event in metabolic control, and thus it is important for readers to understand its utility and management. It also discusses several new techniques for the screening and diagnosis of hypoglycemia.

We would like to thank the authors for their excellent contributions to this book. We are also thankful to our author service manager at IntechOpen for assisting at every step of the book's publication.

Alok Raghav
Multidisciplinary Research Unit,
GSVM Medical College,
Kanpur, India

Section 1

Introduction to Hypoglycemia

Chapter 1

Hypoglycemic Activity of Plant-Derived Traditional Preparations Associated with Surinamese from African, Hindustani, Javanese, and Chinese Origin: Potential Efficacy in the Management of Diabetes Mellitus

Dennis R.A. Mans

Abstract

Diabetes represents one of the most frequent causes of morbidity and mortality in the world. Despite the availability of a wide range of efficacious forms of treatment, many patients use traditional (plant-derived) preparations for treating their disease. The Republic of Suriname (South America) has a relatively high prevalence of diabetes. Due to its colonial history, the Surinamese population comprises descendants of all continents, the largest groups being those from enslaved Africans and from indentured laborers from India (called Hindustanis), Indonesia (called Javanese), as well as China. All these groups have preserved their cultural customs including their ethnopharmacological traditions, and are inclined to treat their diseases with plant-based preparations, either alone or together with allopathic medications. This chapter opens with some generalities about diabetes; subsequently provides some information about the history, worldwide epidemiology, diagnosis, types, and treatment of this disorder; then focuses on Suriname, giving some information about its geography, demographics, and economy, as well as the epidemiology of diabetes in the country; then extensively evaluates eight blood-glucose-lowering plants that are mainly associated with the four largest ethnic groups in Suriname by reviewing phytochemical, mechanistic, preclinical, and clinical literature data; and concludes with a consideration of the potential clinical usefulness of the plants against diabetes.

Keywords: diabetes mellitus, medicinal plants, Suriname, preclinical studies, clinical studies, phytochemical composition, pharmacological activity, mechanism of action

1. Introduction

Diabetes mellitus (in short, diabetes) is a metabolic disorder of multiple etiology characterized by sustained hyperglycemia with disturbances of carbohydrate, fat, and protein homeostasis resulting from defects in insulin secretion, insulin action, or both [1]. The defects in insulin secretion are the result of inappropriate functioning of the β cells of the pancreas, while those in insulin action are generally associated with resistance of the peripheral tissues to insulin. In all cases, the end result is a defective availability of insulin [1].

Diabetes usually presents with characteristic symptoms including thirst, polyuria, blurring of vision, as well as weight loss, and when not properly treated, ketoacidosis or a non-ketotic hyperosmotic state that may lead to stupor, coma, and eventually death. However, in many cases, these symptoms are not severe or may even be absent. As a result, potentially critical hyperglycemia may be present long before the diagnosis is made [2]. In the long-term, the effects of diabetes include retinopathy and potential blindness, nephropathy that may lead to renal failure, and/or neuropathy with the risk of foot ulcers, amputation, and features of autonomic dysfunction including sexual debility [2].

This paper first briefly addresses the worldwide epidemiology, diagnosis, and subtypes, as well as the forms of treatment of diabetes; subsequently presents the geography, demographics, and economy, as well as the epidemiology of the disease in the Republic of Suriname; then focuses on the traditional forms of treatment of diabetes in that country, and extensively discusses eight plant species with hypoglycemic properties, two of which are traditionally used against diabetes by each of the four largest ethnic groups in Suriname, namely, the Afro-Surinamese, Hindustani, Javanese, and Chinese; and concludes with the prevision of these plants in the treatment of diabetes.

2. Background

2.1 Worldwide epidemiology

Diabetes is generally considered a major public health threat with a growing burden in many parts of the world. According to the International Diabetes Federation [3], approximately 537 million adults of the 7.9 billion people who populated our globe in 2021, were living with diabetes. This corresponded to about 6.8% of the world population in that year, and this number is anticipated to rise to 643 million by 2030 and 783 million by 2045, i.e., roughly 7.5% and 8.3%, respectively, of the projected sizes of the world population in these years [3]. Furthermore, 541 million adults were at increased risk of developing type 2 diabetes, almost 240 million adults were living with undiagnosed diabetes, more than 1.2 million children and adolescents (0–19 years) with type 1 disease, and 21 million live births (i.e., 1 of 6 live births) were affected by diabetes during pregnancy [3].

Apart from the complications that may accompany diabetes such as nephropathy, retinopathy, neuropathy, and associated foot problems, this disease dramatically increases the risk of cardiovascular problems including coronary artery disease with angina pectoris, heart attack, stroke, and atherosclerosis [4]. Not surprisingly, the costs associated with this disease are astronomical, globally amounting to at least USD 966 billion dollars last year, i.e., 9% of the total worldwide spending on health expenditure in adults [3].

Diabetes was responsible for 6.7 million deaths in 2021 [3]. Notably, this disease occupied in 2019 the 9th position on the list of the top ten causes of death globally, which represented an increase of 70% when compared to 2000 [5]. Diabetes was also responsible for the largest rise in male deaths among the top ten causes, with an 80% increase the mortality rate increasing since 2000 [5]. In that year, it was in 10th place of the leading causes of death in high-income countries and in 9th and 6th place of those in low- and middle-income, and upper-middle-income countries, respectively [5]. It has been estimated that 3 of 4 adults suffering from diabetes are living in low- and middle-income countries [3]. This has largely been attributed to these countries rapidly adopting a Western lifestyle including Western dietary patterns (particularly during adolescence), reduced physical activity, and increased stress [6, 7]. The Caribbean, for instance, has the highest age-adjusted prevalence of diabetes in the world at 10.8% [6], with some countries in that region reporting prevalence rates of 18% [7]. This is considerably higher than both the worldwide prevalence and the prevalence in South and Central America, which is about 7.5% [6]. Indeed, diabetes particularly represents a major public health threat for developing countries.

2.2 Diagnosis and subtypes

The most recent diagnostic criteria for diabetes are those from the American Diabetes Association, involving glycosylated hemoglobin (HbA1c) blood levels ≥6.5%, fasting plasma glucose levels ≥126 mg/dL or 7.0 mmol/L, 2-h plasma glucose levels ≥200 mg/dL or 11.1 mmol/L during an oral glucose tolerance test, and/or classic symptoms of hyperglycemia or hyperglycemic crisis with random plasma glucose ≥200 mg/dL or 11.1 mmol/L [8]. Depending on the severity and the etiologic background, diabetes is distinguished in the clinical categories prediabetes, type 1 diabetes, type 2 diabetes, gestational diabetes, and other subtypes such as those caused by genetic defects in cell function, genetic defects in insulin, disorders of the pancreas, and the use of certain drugs [9].

Individuals with prediabetes have elevated blood sugar levels which are, however, not sufficiently high to qualify for the diagnosis of "diabetes" [10]. Many such individuals are not aware of their condition, but prediabetes is an important predisposing factor for 2 diabetes as well as heart disease [10]. Type 1 diabetes (also referred to as insulin-dependent diabetes and previously called juvenile-onset diabetes) is most common in childhood and early adulthood [11]. It is an autoimmune condition involving own antibodies attacking and destroying the pancreatic β-cells, eventually resulting in absolute insulin deficiency [11]. Type 1 diabetes can cause a multitude of health problems which are mostly related to retinopathy, neuropathy, and nephropathy as well as a high risk of heart disease and stroke [11].

Type 2 diabetes is also known as non-insulin-dependent, insulin-resistant, and adult-onset diabetes, but has become more common in children and teens over the past 20 years, largely because more young people are overweight or obese [12]. Currently, about 90% of individuals with diabetes have type 2 [12]. In patients with type 2 diabetes, the pancreas either produces insufficient amounts of insulin, or the target tissues in the body (particularly fat, liver, and muscle) do not properly respond or do not respond at all to insulin [12]. Although type 2 diabetes is often milder than type 1, it can cause major health complications including retinopathy, neuropathy, and nephropathy, as well as an increased risk of heart disease and stroke [12].

Gestational diabetes occurs in 1–14% of all pregnancies depending on the population and the method of assessment [13]. This condition is a form of insulin resistance that usually manifests in middle or late pregnancy as a result of progressive changes in the metabolism of the pregnant woman including hormonal levels such as those of cortisol and estrogen [13]. Gestational diabetes usually ceases after birth, but up to 10% of women suffering from this condition are at risk to develop type 2 diabetes in a later stage of their life and carry the risk of unusual weight gain of the baby before birth necessitating cesarean section, respiratory problems of the newborn at birth, as well as a higher risk of obesity and type 2 diabetes of the child at an older age [13].

An estimated 1–5% of cases of diabetes are caused by conditions other than those mentioned above, including those with a genetic background and those that are non-genetically related. Types of diabetes with a genetic background are neonatal diabetes [14] and maturity-onset diabetes in the young [15], Wolfram syndrome-related (type 1) diabetes [16], and cystic fibrosis-related (type 1) diabetes [17]. Types of diabetes with a non-genetic background are, among others, chronic pancreatitis-associated diabetes, which is usually caused by extensive damage to the exocrine tissue of the pancreas [18], brittle diabetes, which primarily affects patients with type 1 diabetes and manifests as frequent and severe fluctuations in blood glucose levels [19], and Cushing's syndrome-related diabetes [20].

2.3 Treatment

Since the early days of diabetes treatment involving insulin replacement therapy [21], this treatment modality has taken considerable strides in terms of devices for administration and formulations with variability in onset, peak, and duration of action. Some examples of injectable devices are single-use syringes, insulin pens, insulin jet injectors, and external insulin pumps [22]. As well, the biochemical and pharmacological properties of endogenous insulin have been modified in order to produce insulins that give a constant low basal level of insulin or lower insulin spikes in response to meals so as to attain less hypoglycemia and improvement of postprandial glucose control. This has resulted in rapid-acting, short-acting, intermediate-acting, long-acting, and ultra-long-acting insulin preparations, as well as certain mixtures and concentrated formulations [23]. The next steps in insulin therapy will likely involve "smart" insulins which will be delivered according to an endogenous glucose-sensing feedback mechanism, novel needle-free insulin delivery devices for subcutaneous administrations, and alternative routes of insulin delivery such as pulmonary, nasal, buccal, oral, and transdermal routes [24].

Furthermore, a host of antidiabetic remedies other than insulin have become available [25, 26]. These drugs can be classified according to their mechanism of action as insulinotropic or non-insulinotropic, and they are given as a monotherapy or in certain combinations without or with insulin, usually for type 2 diabetes [25, 26]. The insulinotropic agents depend on their actions on residual β-cell function and stimulate the secretion of insulin from the pancreatic β-cells. They include the sulfonylureas (such as tolbutamide and glibenclamide), the meglitinide analogs (such as repaglinide), the glucose-dependent glucagon-like peptide-1 receptor agonists (GLP-1 agonists) or incretin mimetics (such as exenatide), and the dipeptidyl peptidase 4 inhibitors (DPP-4 inhibitors) or gliptins (such as sitagliptin). The non-insulinotropic agents are effective in patients with non-functional pancreatic β-cells. They include the biguanides (such as metformin), the sodium-glucose co-transporter-2 inhibitors (SGLT-2 inhibitors) or gliflozins (such as dapagliflozin), the thiazolidinediones or glitazones (such as rosiglitazone), the α-glucosidase inhibitors (such as acarbose), and the amylin agonist analogs (such as pramlintide). Almost all these antidiabetic drugs are taken orally, except for the GLP-1 agonists and the amylin agonist analogs which are injectable. Of note, several new drug combinations such as metformin in combination with an SGLT2 inhibitor and a DPP4 inhibitor are now undergoing clinical evaluation [26].

3. The Republic of Suriname

3.1 Geography, demographics, and economy

The Republic of Suriname is located on the northeastern Atlantic coast of South America, adjacent to French Guiana, Brazil, and Guyana (**Figure 1**). The country has a land area of about 165,000 km^2 that can be distinguished into a northern narrow low-land coastal plain that harbors the capital city Paramaribo as well as other urbanized areas, a broad but sparsely inhabited savannah belt, and a southern forested hinterland that comprises about three-quarters of its surface and largely consists of dense, pristine, and highly biodiverse tropical rain forest (**Figure 1**). Roughly 80% of the population of about 600,000 lives in the urbanized northern coastal zone while the remaining 20% populates the rural and interior savannas and hinterlands [27].

Suriname is renowned for its ethnic, religious, and cultural diversity, harboring various Amerindian tribes, the original inhabitants of the country; Afro-Surinamese, comprising the descendants of enslaved Africans brought in between the sixteenth and the 19th century who fled the plantations and settled in the country's hinterland (called Maroons) as well as those from mixed Black and White origin (called Creoles); the descendants from contract workers from India (called Hindustanis); Java, Indonesia (called Javanese); and China, all of whom arrived between the second half of the 19th century and the first half of the 20th century; the descendants from a number of European countries; and more recently, immigrants from various Latin American and Caribbean countries including Brazil, Guyana, French Guiana, Haiti, etc. [27]. The largest ethnic groups in the country are the Afro-Surinamese (Creoles and Maroons), Hindustanis, Javanese, and Chinese, accounting for 37.4, 27.4, 15.7, and 7.3%, respectively, of the total population [27]. All ethnic groups have largely preserved their own specific identity, making Suriname one of the culturally most diverse countries in the world [28].

Suriname is situated on the Guiana Shield, a Precambrian geological formation estimated to be 1.7 billion years old and one of the regions with the largest expanse of undisturbed tropical rain forest in the world with a very high animal and plant biodiversity [29]. The high mineral density contributes to its ranking as the 17th richest country in the world in terms of natural resources and development potential [30]. Suriname's most important economic means of support are crude oil drilling, gold mining, agriculture, fisheries, forestry, as well as ecotourism [30]. These activities have substantially contributed to the gross domestic income in 2020 of about USD 3 billion and the average per capita income in that year of USD 4920 [30, 31]. This positions Suriname on the World Bank's list of upper-middle-income economies [31].

3.2 Epidemiology of diabetes in Suriname

As observed in many low- and middle-income countries [32], increasingly more Surinamese are adapting to a Western lifestyle. Indeed, only about half of the

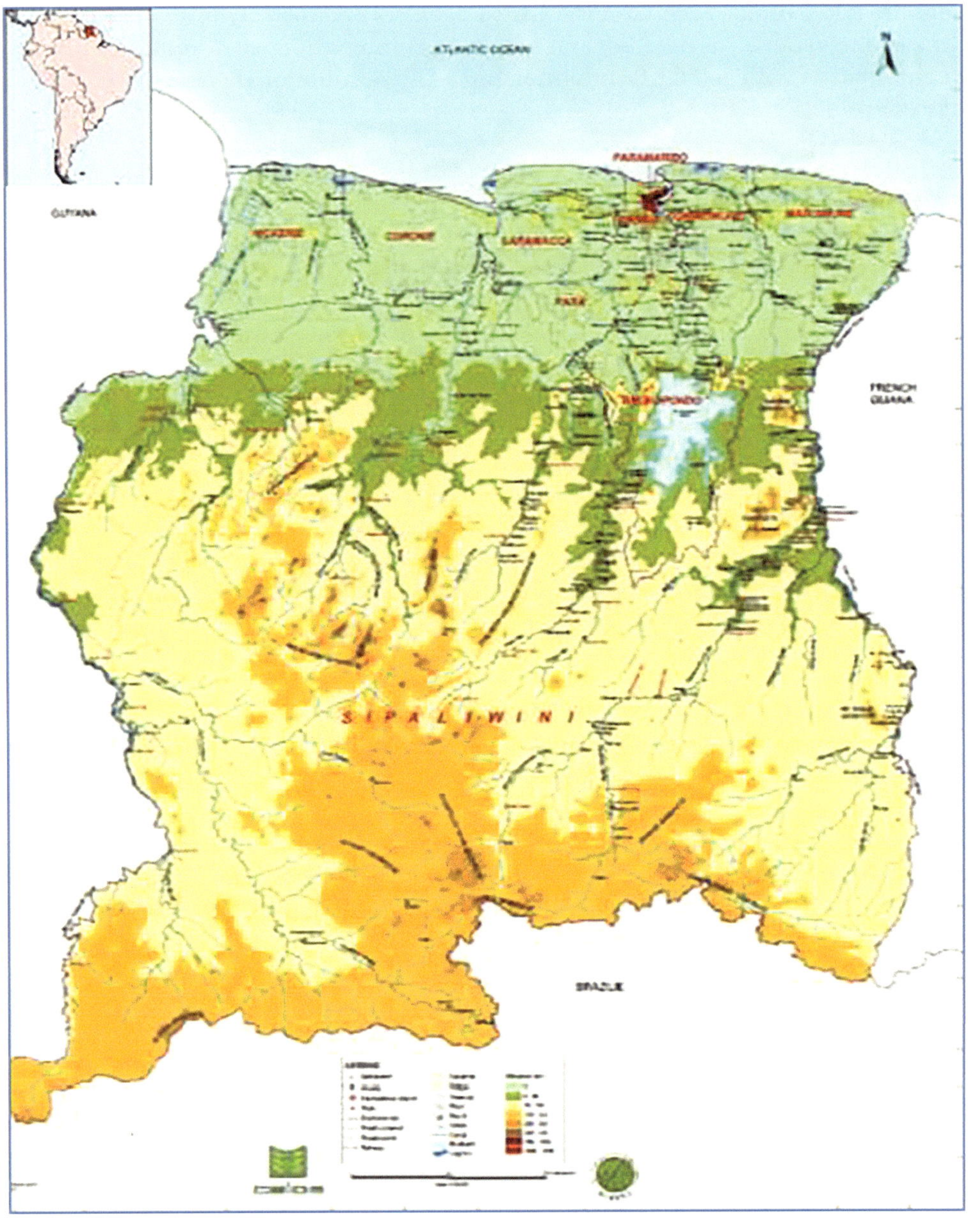

Figure 1.
Map of the Republic of Suriname, showing the southern interior or hinterland (yellow-brown); the savanna belt (dark green); and the northern coastal plain (light green) (from: https://images.app.goo.gl/Gr8fsdAaoqp3LpVn7). Insert: the position of Suriname (red) in South America (from: https://images.app.goo.gl/i4KL8WisoWW8TFmS9).

country's overall population meets the levels for physical activity recommended by the World Health Organization [33]; almost three-quarters of school children aged 13–15 years have less than 1 h of physical activity per day and 81% have too high calorie intake [34]; about 1 of 5 adults is overweight and approximately 1 of 15 is obese [35]; the average tobacco and alcohol consumption per capita in individuals of 15 years and older is unacceptably high [34]; the overall estimated prevalence of the metabolic syndrome is 39.2% [36]; and more than 25% of adults has a raised blood pressure [36]. Notably, with almost 200 deaths per year, diabetes is the 4th principal cause of mortality in Suriname, after cardiovascular diseases, external causes, and cancer [37].

Accordingly, the Suriname Health Study—the first nationwide study on non-communicable disease risk factors in Suriname [38]—reported an overall prevalence of prediabetes in the country of about 7.4% and diabetes of 13.0% [39]. The latter value is well in agreement with that of 12.7% recently estimated for Suriname by the International Diabetic Federation [3]. This figure represents a substantial increase with respect to that of 8.9% in 2011 and is likely to rise to 14.0% by 2030 and 14.6% in 2045 [3]. Accordingly, the health expenditures for diabetes in Suriname—estimated at about USD 63.5 million in 2021—are anticipated to reach USD 70.1 million in 2030 and USD 80.1 million in 2045 [3].

4. Traditional forms of treatment of diabetes in Suriname

As mentioned above, the different ethnic groups in Suriname have largely preserved their cultural heritage including their specific (plant-based) traditional customs [28]. This has resulted in the many forms of traditional medicine practiced in the country including those based on traditional Indigenous medicine, traditional African medicine, Indian Ayurveda and Unani, Javanese Jamu, traditional Chinese medicine, and several other forms of complementary and alternative medicine [28]. The botanical knowledge and the plant materials for establishing and maintaining these systems probably came from several sources, including previous acquaintance with useful plants, new information about the local flora from the Indigenous peoples, and/or the selection of potentially valuable plants by trial and error [28, 40].

That the enslaved Africans and Asian indentured laborers were familiar with certain plants they encountered in Suriname, is presumably for an important part attributable to the Columbian Exchange in the fifteenth and sixteenth centuries, when many plants—as well as animals, people, commodities, and diseases—had been transferred from the Old World (Europe, Asia, and Africa) to the New World (the Americas) and vice versa [41, 42]. As a result, when the newcomers arrived in Suriname in the second half of the seventeenth century on, they immediately recognized many New World food crops and medicinal plants which were indigenous to their homeland [43, 44] or which had been introduced into their homeland more than 100 years before [42, 45]. A few examples are several yam species in the genus *Dioscorea* (Dioscoreaceae), and a number of ginger species in the plant family Zingiberaceae [43, 44], as well as okra (*Abelmoschus esculentus* (L.) Moench; Malvaceae), bitter melon (*Momordica charantia* L.; Cucurbitaceae), and eggplant (*Solanum melongena* L.; Solanaceae) [42, 45]. In addition, the enslaved Africans had carried medicinal plants such as the tamarind *Tamarindus indica* L. 1753 (Fabaceae) with them in order to fight diseases such as fever, diarrhea, and worm infections on the slave ships [46, 47].

Furthermore, the Maroons—but perhaps also individuals who arrived in Suriname after them—acquired new knowledge about useful plants through contact with the indigenous peoples and by trial and error. For instance, the application of the paste from the ground orange-red seeds from the annatto *Bixa orellana* L. (Bixaceae) as an insect repellent [48], and that of preparation from the leaves from the ink plant *Renealmia alpinia* (Rottb.) Maas (1975) (Zingiberaceae) as a remedy for snakebites

Plant family	Plant species (vernacular name in English; in Surinamese or language of origin)	Part(s) mostly used
Acanthaceae	*Ruellia tuberosa* L. (minnieroot; watrakanu)	Root
Amaranthaceae	*Gomphrena globosa* L. (globe amaranth; stanvaste)	Leaf and flower
Myrtaceae	*Syzygium cumini* (L.) Skeels (jambolan; jamún)	Seed
Rutaceae	*Aegle marmelos* (L.) Corrêa (bael; bhel)	Fruit
Acanthaceae	*Strobilanthes crispa* (L.) Blume (black face general; ketji beling)	Leaf
Clusiaceae	*Garcinia mangostana* L. (mangosteen; manggis)	Fruit
Araliaceae	*Panax notoginseng* (Burkill) F.H.Chen (Chinese ginseng; san-qi)	Root and rhizome
Lauraceae	*Cinnamomum cassia* (L.) J.Presl. (Chinese cassia; guān guì)	Bark

Table 1.
Plants with hypoglycemic activity addressed in this chapter, parts mostly used, and mode of preparation.

[49] stems from Indigenous knowledge. And the selection of potentially useful plants by trial and error has not only led to fatalities by poisonous plants but also to the use of such plants (like the jackass breadnut *Clibadium surinamense* L. (Asteraceae)) as arrow and fish poisons [50].

The next sections address in detail eight plant species with hypoglycemic properties, two of which are traditionally used against diabetes by each of the four largest ethnic groups in Suriname (the Afro-Surinamese, Hindustani, Javanese, and Chinese). The plants and herbal products associated with the three former groups have been selected on the basis of the number of times they have been mentioned in comprehensive publications on Surinamese medicinal plants [51–55]. Such documents are not available for plants and herbal products related to the Surinamese-Chinese. Therefore, information about anti-diabetic substances associated with this group has been obtained from a Surinamese-Chinese pharmacist, and from the imports of herbal products from the People's Republic of China by Surinamese-Chinese importers and distributors. Relevant information about the plants is given in **Table 1**. Preclinical and clinical indications for their hypoglycemic effect, as well as their presumed bioactive constituent(s) and mechanism(s) of action, are in detail addressed hereunder and have been summarized in **Table 2**.

5. Plants with hypoglycemic properties associated with Surinamese from African origin

5.1 Acanthaceae: *Ruellia tuberosa* L.

The minnieroot *R. tuberosa* L. (Acanthaceae) (**Figure 2**) is probably native to Central America, the West Indies, and northern South America including Suriname, but has become naturalized in many other tropical countries throughout the world. It is popularly known as "cracker plant" in English-speaking regions and as "watra kanu" ("water canon") in Surinamese-Creole because of the loud crack emitted when the ripe fruits in a pod with the black seeds burst open on contact with water, hurdling the seeds away. The whole plant as well as leaf, seed, and root

Plant species	Preclinical evidence	Clinical evidence	Presumed pharmacologically active constituent(s)	Presumed mechanism(s) of hypoglycemia
R. tuberosa	Yes	No	Triterpenoids and flavonoids	Antioxidant activity; inhibition of digestive enzymes
G. globosa	Yes	No	Flavonoids	Increased insulin secretion; improved insulin resistance and sensitivity; decreased gluconeogenesis; inhibition of digestive enzymes; antioxidant activity
S. cumini	Yes	Limited	Phenolic compounds such as ferulic acid; flavonoids such as kaempferol and myrecetin; alkaloids such as jambosine; glycosides such as jambolin	Antioxidant activity; increased PPAR expression; inhibition of digestive enzymes
A. marmelos	Yes	Limited	Phenylethyl cinnamides such as anhydroaegeline	Increased insulin secretion; increased glucose uptake; inhibition of digestive enzymes
S. crispa	Yes	No	Several phenolic compounds	Antioxidant activity
G. mangostana	Yes	No	Xanthones such as garcimangostin A, proanthocyanidins, and mangostins	Antioxidant activity; inhibition of digestive enzymes
P. notoginseng	Yes	Limited	Dammarane saponines such as notoginsenosides	Increased glycogenesis; increased insulin secretion; improved insulin resistance and sensitivity; increased GLUT4 expression; antioxidant activity
C. cassia	Yes	Limited	Phenylpropanoids such as cinnamaldehyde	Antioxidant activity; inhibition of digestive enzymes; increased glycogenesis; improved insulin resistance and sensitivity

Table 2.
Preclinical and clinical evidence for antidiabetic activity of eight commonly used plants in Suriname for the traditional treatment of diabetes mellitus, the presumed key active constituent(s) in the plants, and their presumed mechanism of action.

are used in various traditional medical systems including those from the Afro-Surinamese, for preparing medicines for treating, among others, stomach ache, indigestion, constipation; problems of the urinary tract; eczema and skin eruptions; headache, fever, influenza, bronchitis, asthma, pneumonia, and whooping cough; hypertension and heart ailments; malaria; joint pain; venereal diseases; vaginal

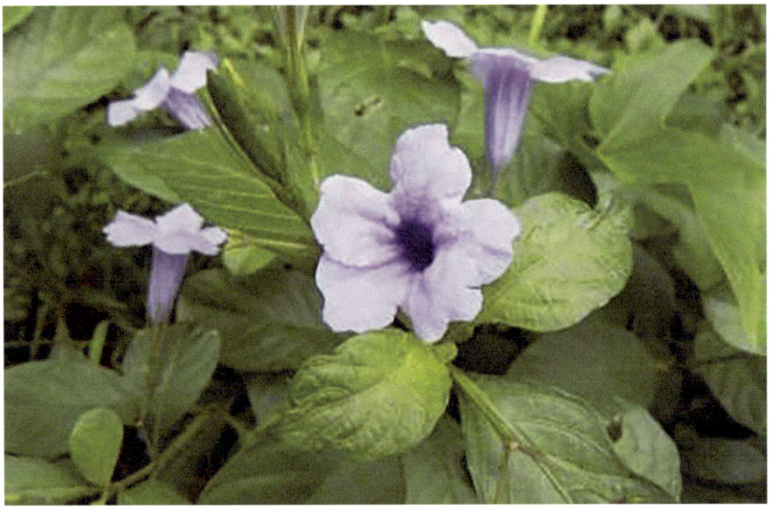

Figure 2.
Flowers of the minnieroot or watrakanu Ruellia tuberosa *L. (Acanthaceae) (from: https://images.app.goo.gl/JjLuHr66h8rca2c67).*

discharge; and reduced sexual performance or pleasure [56, 57]. Some of these uses are supported by the results from pharmacological studies reporting, among others, gastroprotective, antiurolithiatic, antimicrobial, anti-inflammatory, larvicidal, and antifertility activities of the plant [56, 57]. These activities have been associated with the presence in the plant of certain alkaloids, triterpenoids, saponins, sterols, and flavonoids [58].

In Suriname and various other Caribbean countries, an infusion or decoction of *R. tuberosa* root is also used against diabetes [52, 54, 55]. So far, however, no clinical studies have been carried out to corroborate this use. Still, there is ample preclinical evidence for the antidiabetic activity of this plant. Firstly, extracts and fractions of several of its parts elicited clear hypoglycemic effects in normal and alloxan- or streptozotocin-induced rodent models of diabetes [59–63]. The decline in blood glucose was accompanied by a decrease in HbA1c levels and an amelioration of abnormal hepatic detoxification function [62] as well as a decrease in insulin resistance [63]. Furthermore, the *R. tuberosa* preparations led to substantial improvements in the histopathology of kidney, pancreas, and liver of the diabetic animals [64, 65]. The extract also caused a notable improvement in glucose uptake in insulin-resistant mouse C2C12 myoblasts [63], supporting that it may overcome insulin resistance in skeletal muscle cells. The hypoglycemic activity (of root preparations) was comparable to that found for tolbutamide [59] and glibenclamide [60].

The hypoglycemic activity of *R. tuberosa* may be associated with the antioxidant properties of some of its constituents, as shown by the notable 2,2-diphenyl-1-picrylhydrazyl (DPPH)-scavenging activity of preparations from the plant [59]. Furthermore, the administration of a root extract led to an increase in catalase and superoxide dismutase activities as well as a decrease in malondialdehyde levels (a measure of lipid peroxidation) in induced hypercholesterolemic rats and streptozotocin-induced rats [62, 64–66]. *R. tuberosa* preparations also displayed a relatively high content of total phenolic compounds and flavonoids [59, 60, 67], some of which have been shown to protect against the oxidative stress that is considered an important contributing factor to the initiation and development of many diseases including diabetes [68, 69]. The hypoglycemic effects were accompanied by a decrease in blood concentrations of cholesterol, triglycerides, LDL-c, and VLDL, and an increase in HDL-c in various animal models [60, 66, 70]. These observations compared favorably with glibenclamide [60, 70].

The results from animal and *in vitro* studies suggest that the hypoglycemic actions of *R. tuberosa* could also be associated with the inhibition of α-amylase activity [61] and/or α-glucosidase activity [71]. Thus, preparations from this plant may be useful for controlling postprandial hyperglycemia by preventing the digestion of carbohydrates and delaying the increase in blood glucose [72]. Compounds in *R. tuberosa* that may be responsible for its α-amylase and α-glucosidase inhibitory activity are the pentacyclic triterpenoid betulin [61] and certain phenolic compounds including several flavonoids [67, 71, 73], respectively. This is consistent with the identification in the plant of triterpenoids and flavonoids [67], the hypoglycemic effects of these substances [59], and the implication of antioxidant activities in their blood glucose-lowering capacity [68, 69].

5.2 Amaranthaceae: *Gomphrena globosa* L.

The globe amaranth *Gomphrena globosa* L. (Amaranthaceae) (**Figure 3**) is an annual herb that grows to a height of 1 meter and that presumably originates from Asia but is now cultivated as an ornamental in many tropical and subtropical parts of the world including Suriname. *G. globosa* produces small and inconspicuous flowers but vividly colored round-shaped flower inflorescences that range from pink to red and purple in some cultivars. The flower inflorescences do not readily wither and retain their shape and color after drying and are therefore used in long-lasting garlands. This characteristic is reflected by the Surinamese-Creole vernacular names “stanvaste” and “stanfasti” for the plant, meaning “lasting” or “steadfast.” For this reason, the more fanatical supporters of the mostly Creole social-democratic political party “National Party of Suriname” have claimed *G. globosa* as their (unofficial) symbol.

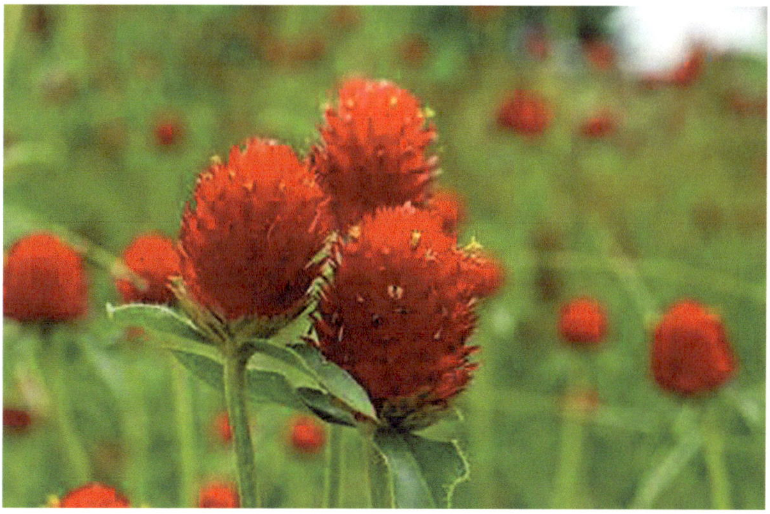

Figure 3.
Flower inflorescences of the globe amaranth or stanvaste Gomphrena globosa *L. (Amaranthaceae) (from: https://images.app.goo.gl/fxEMirfxTQZPZhENA).*

The flowers of *G. globosa* also serve as a source of betacyanins for use as a (red-violet) colorant in the food, cosmetic, and pharmaceutical industry [74]. Betacyanins are a subclass of betalain pigments, aromatic indole derivatives that are synthesized from tyrosine to produce glycosides consisting of a sugar and a colored portion [75]. One of the most notable betalains is betanin or beetroot red in the beet *Beta vulgaris* L. (Amaranthaceae) [75]. Betalains are chemically distinct from anthocyanins or flavonoids but replace anthocyanin pigments in plants of the order Caryophyllales (that includes *G. globosa*) and in certain fungi [75]. In plants, they probably attract pollinators and seed dispersers and act as antioxidants, providing protection against harmful reactive oxygen species [75].

Parts of *Gomphrena* species are used in various countries for preparing traditional remedies. A few indications are oliguria and other urinary conditions; reproductive problems; microbial and parasitic infections; skin diseases and wounds; fever and respiratory disorders such as bronchitis and whooping cough; gastrointestinal disorders such as jaundice; high cholesterol; as well as hypertension [76, 77]. The potential therapeutic usefulness against these conditions is supported by, among others, the antioxidant, anti-inflammatory, analgesic, antimicrobial, and cytotoxic activities of preparations from the plant [76, 77]. These pharmacological activities have mainly been associated with the betalains but also with certain saponins, tannins, flavonoids, and alkaloids in the plant [76–78].

G. globosa is also a popular traditional remedy against diabetes in various parts of the world [76, 77]. In Suriname, an infusion of its leaf and flower is used to lower excessively high blood glucose levels [52]. There are no studies with diabetics to back this custom, but there is some preclinical support for hypoglycemic activity of this plant. For instance, a crude methanol extract from the whole plant as well as an n-hexane fraction therefrom showed meaningful hypoglycemic activity in Swiss-albino mice subjected to a glucose tolerance test [79]. The hypoglycemic activity was comparable to that of glibenclamide [79]. As well, repeated administration of a leaf ethanolic extract lowered blood glucose in alloxan-induced hyperglycemic Wistar rats [80].

Rather than to the betalains, the hypoglycemic activity of *G. globosa* has been attributed to one or more flavonoids in the plant [76–78, 80]. These compounds have been suggested to lower blood sugar in laboratory animals by stimulating the secretion of insulin by the pancreatic β-cells, the utilization of glucose by the body tissues, and/or the decrease of hepatic gluconeogenesis [80]. In a series of *in vitro* studies, an ethanolic leaf extract of *G. globosa* exhibited meaningful α-amylase inhibitory activity [81], suggesting that eliminating postprandial blood glucose spikes was also involved in its antidiabetic effects. The leaf extract also displayed notable *in vitro* antiglycation and antioxidant activity [81, 82], suggesting that antioxidant mechanisms may also contribute to the antidiabetic activity of the plant [68, 69].

6. Plants with hypoglycemic properties associated with Surinamese from Hindustani origin

6.1 Myrtaceae: *Syzygium cumini* (L.) Skeels

The jambolan *Syzygium cumini* (L.) Skeels (Myrtaceae) (**Figure 4**), called "jamún" by Surinamese-Hindustani, is native to the Indian subcontinent but is now grown in various tropical and subtropical regions worldwide. It has presumably

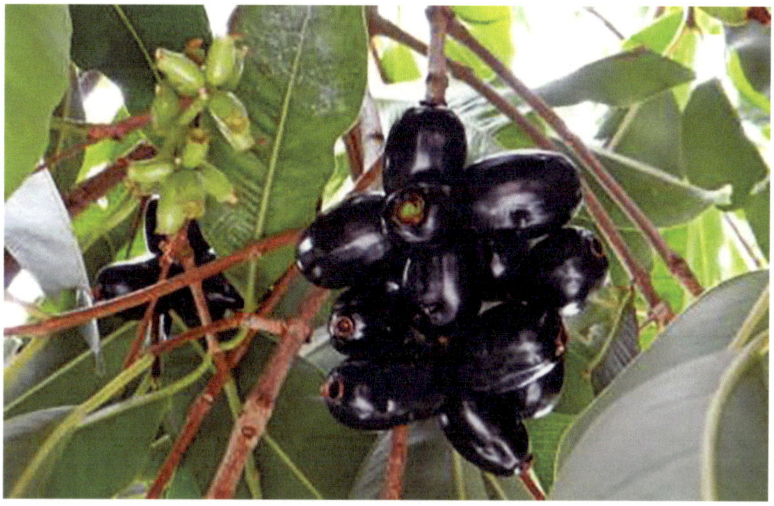

Figure 4.
Fruits of the jambolan or jamún Syzygium cumini *(L.) Skeels (Myrtaceae) (from: https://images.app.goo.gl/AXjEW9A1nFFgi1nDA).*

brought to Suriname by Hindustani indentured laborers at the end of the 19th and the beginning of the 20th century. This is reflected in the Surinamese vernacular "kulidroifi," meaning "the grape from the coolies," in reference to the then European pejorative for Hindustani indentured laborers. *S. cumini* produces ovoid, edible fruits that are green when unripe and become pink, then crimson red, and finally purplish-black as they mature. The sweet and mildly sour-tasting and astringent fruits are eaten raw, and can also be made into juices, wines, jellies, sorbets, syrups, jams, sauces, or fruit salads.

All parts of *S. cumini*, but particularly its bark, leaf, seed, and fruit, have since long been used in Indian Ayurveda and Unani as well as various other traditional medical systems for treating, among others, coughing, asthma, and bronchitis; stomachache, dyspepsia, colic, diarrhea, dysentery, liver problems, and hemorrhoids; ringworm, piles, pimples, skin blemishes, and acne; various types of inflammation; fatigue and strain; blisters in the mouth and weak teeth and gums; cancer; and diabetes [83, 84]. In Suriname, a tea or coffee-like beverage prepared from macerated *S. cumini* seeds is also used against the symptoms of diabetes, a custom that probably originates from the Hindustanis [53, 55].

Some of the traditional uses of *S. cumini* may be accounted for by alkaloids such as jambosine, glycosides such as glycoside jambolin, as well as phenolic compounds including gallic acid, caffeic acid, and ellagic acid; flavonoids such as quercetin, myricetin, and kaempferol; anthocyanins such as delphinidin-3,5-O-diglucoside, petunidin-3,5-O-diglucoside, and malvidin-3,5-O-diglucoside; and tannins such as ellagitannins [83, 84]. These compounds as well as crude *S. cumini* preparations displayed, among others, antioxidant, antimicrobial, antimalarial, anti-inflammatory, analgesic, and anticancer activities [85, 86].

There is also substantial pharmacological evidence to support the broad traditional use of *S. cumini*—particularly with its seed—for treating diabetes. Thus, administration of the seed powder or various types of extracts from the seed or the seed kernel, led to a decrease in blood glucose levels in alloxan- or streptozotocin-induced rodents [87–90], an increase in glucose tolerance [91], a reduction in insulin resistance [92], positive effects on pancreatic islet cell regeneration [93, 94], and an improvement in blood lipid profiles [87, 90, 91, 95]. Comparable, although less pronounced results were obtained with *S. cumini* root, stem bark, leaf, and fruit preparations [92, 96, 97].

The blood-glucose-lowering activity of *S. cumini* may involve the mitigation of the oxidative stress associated with the development of diabetes [68, 69]. This can be inferred from preclinical studies showing an increase in antioxidant defenses and a decrease in lipid peroxidation in animal models of diabetes treated with a seed preparation [98–100]. Candidates in the seed with such antioxidant properties are phenolic compounds such as ferulic acid [101–103] and flavonoids such as kaempferol and myrecetin [98, 99]. The hypoglycemic activity of *S. cumini* may also be attributable to its capacity to activate and increase the expression of the genes encoding for peroxisome proliferators activated receptors gamma and alpha (PPARγ and PPARα) in the liver, increasing insulin sensitivity of the target tissues [95]. In addition, various *in vitro* and animal studies with *S. cumini* seed and leaf preparations showed an inhibitory effect on α-amylase and α-glucosidase activity, suggesting that these substances lowered postprandial blood glucose [104–106]. This effect may be ascribed to the alkaloid jambosine and the glycoside jambolin in the seed [83].

So far, only a relative handful clinical studies have been conducted on the antidiabetic efficacy of *S. cumini* in diabetics [107]. Unfortunately, the results from these studies were inconclusive, some suggesting that the preparations helped control blood sugar levels whereas others did not show any improvement [107]. For instance, the administration of seed preparations to patients with (severe) type 2 diabetes reportedly led to promising reductions in fasting and postprandial blood glucose levels [108–114] as well as less polyphagia, polyuria, polydipsia, and fatigue [109, 113]. However, a dried and powdered leaf decoction did not elicit an effect on blood glucose levels in either non-diabetic young volunteers submitted to a glucose blood tolerance test [115] or type 2 diabetic patients [116].

6.2 Rutaceae: *Aegle marmelos* (L.) Corrêa

Aegle marmelos (L.) Corrêa (Rutaceae) (**Figure 5**), commonly known as bael or golden apple, is the only member of the genus *Aegle*. It is probably native to India and has spread to nearby countries such as Bangladesh, Sri Lanka, and Nepal as well as more distant tropical and subtropical countries including Suriname. In the latter country, it has presumably been introduced by Hindustani indentured laborers around the turn of the 20th century. *A. marmelos* is also called "bhel" or "bill patr," meaning "the flavorful fruit with the hard shell" [53], in reference to its globose or slightly pear-shaped fruit of 5–12 cm in diameter with a hard-wooden, yellow to gray-greenish shell and an aromatic, pale-orange, sticky, sweet and resinous pulp. *A. marmelos* has presumably been cultivated for its fruit since 800 BC that can be consumed fresh, prepared as lemonade, or processed into candy, toffee, pulp powder, or nectar after being dried. The leaves and small shoots are eaten as salad greens. The alkaloid aegeline in leaf and fruit has been marketed as the dietary supplement OxyELITE Pro® for weight loss and muscle building [117]. However, it has been withdrawn from the market due to its association with potentially fatal liver damage [117].

All parts of *A. marmelos*—but particularly its fruit and leaf—have a long medical use in Indian Ayurveda and other traditional medical systems [118, 119]. Some indications are chronic diarrhea, dysentery, dyspepsia, peptic ulcers, constipation, and malabsorption; wheezing cough and bronchial spasms; microbial, viral, and parasitic infections; fever and rheumatism; neurological diseases; and cancer [118, 119].

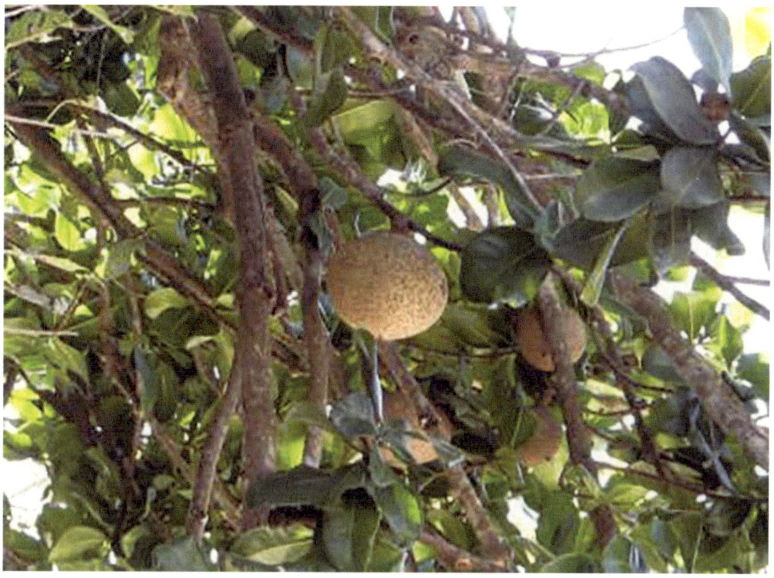

Figure 5.
Fruits of the bael tree or bhel Aegle marmelos *(L.) Corrêa (Rutaceae) (from: https://images.app.goo.gl/SqaKhRAEja9Se8Rx8.*

Scientific studies have validated many of the ethnomedical uses of *A. marmelos*, showing antidiarrheal, gastroprotective, bronchospasmolytic, anti-inflammatory, analgesic, antimicrobial, antiviral, as well as anticancer and chemopreventive effects [120, 121]. These pharmacological activities could partially be attributed to alkaloids in the plant other than aegeline, as well as phenolic compounds, flavonoids, tannins, monoterpenes, and sesquiterpenes, coumarins, saponins, and phytosterols [120, 121].

A. marmelos is also used for the traditional treatment of diabetes in many parts of the world [122, 123] including Suriname [53]. There is ample pharmacological support for this use. Aqueous, methanolic, and ethanolic extracts from fruit, leaf, or an *in vitro* callus culture from a leaf explant produced marked antidiabetic effects in several animal models of diabetes, including normalization of fasting blood glucose level, tolerance to a glucose load, increased serum insulin levels, decreased insulin resistance, improved glucose homeostatic enzymes, and improved blood lipid profile [124–127]. The hypoglycemic activities have been associated with marked antioxidant effects including a decrease in oxidative stress that manifested as a decrease in lipid peroxidation, an increase in the activity of cellular antioxidant mechanisms [128–130], and the regeneration of pancreatic β-cells [126]. These observations are in accordance with the notable antioxidant activity of *A. marmelos* leaf extracts in a DPPH free radical-scavenging assay and a ferric reducing antioxidant power assay [131, 132] as well as in HepG2 cells cultured under glucose-rich conditions [132].

The phytochemicals in the plant that may be involved in its antioxidant activities are the phenolic compound eugenol [133], the furanocoumarin marmesinin [134, 135], the 7-hydroxycoumarin analog umbelliferone β-D-galactopyranoside [136], and the cyclic monoterpene limonene [137]. In addition, *A. marmelos*' antidiabetic activity may be related to the stimulation of insulin release from the pancreas, stimulation of glucose uptake by the skeletal muscles, and lowering of postprandial blood glucose levels. These suggestions are based on the stimulatory effects of

A. marmelos preparations on insulin release by cultured pancreatic islet cells [128] and on glucose uptake by isolated mouse psoas muscle tissue [127], and their substantial inhibitory effects in *in vitro* α-amylase and α-glycosidase assays [138]. At least the α-glycosidase inhibitory activity has been associated with the presence in the leaf of a series of phenylethyl cinnamides, particularly anhydroaegeline [138].

At this moment, only a few clinical studies have been conducted to explore the therapeutic efficacy of *A. marmelos* against diabetes. Leaf preparations given orally to type 2 diabetic patients reportedly lowered levels of fasting blood glucose [139–141], postprandial blood glucose [138–142], and HbA1C [141], along with total blood cholesterol and triglycerides while increasing HDL levels [140, 141]. However, a crossover clinical study evaluating the unripe fruit pulp for 0–21 and 28–49 days with a 7-day wash-out period, did not find an effect on fasting blood glucose [143].

7. Plants with hypoglycemic properties associated with Surinamese from Javanese origin

7.1 Acanthaceae: *Strobilanthes crispa* (L.) Blume

The black face general *Strobilanthes crispa* (L.) Blume (Acanthaceae) (**Figure 6**) is probably native to the Sunda Islands, a group of islands in the Malay Archipelago that includes the Indonesian island of Java. The plant has spread to many south-eastern Asian countries and has presumably been brought to Suriname by Javanese indentured laborers at the end of the 19th century and the beginning of the 20th century [51]. It is a woody spreading shrub that carries yellow-colored flowers, attains a height of 50 cm to 1 m, and can be found on riverbanks and abandoned fields. *S. crispa* is known as "ketji beling" in Surinamese-Javanese, "etji" meaning "very bad" or "vile"

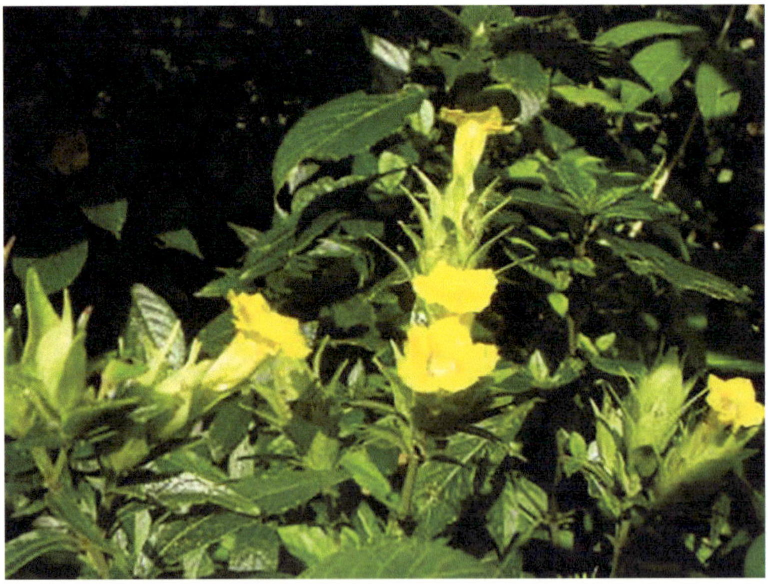

Figure 6.
Leaves and flowers of the black face general or ketji beling Strobilanthes crispa *(L.) Blume (Acanthaceae) (from: https://images.app.goo.gl/AMKPw44x1JPFUqnn9).*

and "beling" meaning "broken glass" or "shards" which probably refers to the very rough texture of both surfaces of the leaves. Nevertheless, this part of the plant is eaten as a vegetable.

In addition, *S. crispa* is used in Indonesian and Malaysian traditional medicine as a diuretic, antilithic, laxative, and anticancer agent [144, 145]. Some of these folk medicinal uses are supported by data from pharmacological studies with leaf preparations showing antimicrobial, antioxidant, antiulcerogenic, anticancer, anti-angiogenic, acetylcholinesterase-inhibitory, and wound healing activity [146–148]. Phytochemical investigations have revealed that *S. crispa* leaf contains polyphenols, flavonoids, catechins, alkaloids, caffeine, and tannins, all of which are known to elicit some of these as well as other pharmacological activities [146–148].

S. crispa has also been used for a long time in particularly Indonesian and Malaysian folk medicine as an ingredient of popular jamus for lowering elevated blood sugar levels [149]. As a result, some products prepared from the leaf of the plant have recently entered the health-food market as antidiabetic nutraceuticals in the form of sachets containing the raw crude powder (fermented and unfermented) for preparing a tea, as an additive in coffee, or as capsules for oral intake [150]. So far, no clinical data are available on the safety and side effects of the long-term use of these products, but several pharmacological studies reported that they do not exert acute toxicity [151, 152].

Like Indonesians and other peoples from south-eastern Asian countries, Surinamese-Javanese use tea from *S. crispa* leaves (alone or together with those from certain other plants) to lower elevated blood sugar levels [51]. This traditional use is supported by the blood-glucose-lowering effects of hot water extracts of fermented and/or unfermented leaf in both normal and streptozotocin-induced diabetic rats [150]. Both preparations also improved lipid profile (total cholesterol, triglyceride, LDL-cholesterol, and HDL-cholesterol) in the animals [150]. *S. crispa* leaf juice given together with a basic diet to streptozotocin-induced diabetic and normal rats produced comparable results, along with significantly increased glutathione peroxidase and superoxide dismutase activities in both groups of animals [153]. Fresh *S. crispa* leaf juice also stimulated the healing of incision wounds on the back of normal and streptozotocin-induced hyperglycemic rats [154]. These observations are in accordance with the stimulatory effects of a topically applied ethanol extract of *S. crispa* leaf on excision wounds in the posterior neck area of normal rats [155] and suggest that this plant may also be useful for treating poorly healing wounds occurring in diabetics.

As mentioned before, plant antioxidants seem to elicit beneficial effects on various aspects of diabetes since oxidative stress probably represents an important contributing factor to the initiation and development of the disease [68, 69]. This is in accordance with the notable antioxidant effects of *S. crispa* preparations in several *in vitro* models of diabetes [148, 156] and their positive effects on endogenous antioxidant mechanisms in diabetic animals such as glutathione peroxidase and superoxide dismutase activities [153]. These effects might be attributed to the abundance of phenolic compounds with antioxidant properties in the plant such as p-hydroxybenzoic acid, p-coumaric acid, caffeic acid, vanillic acid, gentinic acid, ferulic acid, syryngic acid, as well as quercetin, rutin, catechin, myricetin, apigenin, and luteolin [147, 148, 156, 157].

7.2 Clusiaceae: *Garcinia mangostana* L.

The mangosteen *Garcinia mangostana* L. (Clusiaceae) is a tropical evergreen tree that is believed to be native to south-eastern Asia where it is called "manggis" or "manggustan." The exact origin of *G. mangostana* is uncertain but it has been cultivated since ancient times in southern USA, Central America, and north-western South America. It has probably introduced in Suriname by Javanese indentured laborers around the beginning of the 20th century [51]. *G. mangostana* produces round, slightly sweet and sour, flavorful, juicy fruits consisting of fluid-filled vesicles with an inedible, deep reddish-purple colored exocarp when ripe (**Figure 7**). The ripe fruit is eaten raw, incorporated into desserts, added to salads, or made into jams. It is rich in carbohydrates, minerals, vitamins, and various other nutrients [158], and mangosteen-based products are also offered in many parts of the world as "liquid botanical supplements" [159], although the claims of their invigorating properties are being disputed [160]. Interestingly, extracts of the peel have been used for centuries in Indonesia as a natural dye for the brown, dark brown, purple, and red colorings of the characteristic batik textiles [161].

Preparations from *G. mangostana* parts are since ancient times extensively used in traditional south-eastern Asian medicine. A few indications are skin infections, infected wounds, and suppurating sores; dysentery; cystitis; gonorrhea; chronic ulcer, abdominal pain, diarrhea, and dysentery; obesity; as well as cancer [161, 162]. Pharmacological studies have provided support for some of these uses, showing that *G. mangostana* preparations elicit, among others, anti-inflammatory, antibacterial, antiviral, antiprotozoal, antioxidant, anti-obesity, anticancer, and chemopreventive activities [163, 164]. Phytochemical studies have suggested that these activities may particularly be attributed to the high content of polyphenolic compounds in the plant (particularly in pericarp, whole fruit, heartwood, and leaf) such as xanthones, prenylated benzophenone derivatives, flavonoids, anthocyanins, and condensed tannins [163–165]. Xanthones—tricyclic polyphenols consisting of two benzene rings attached through a carbonyl group and oxygen—are the major bioactive constituents in *G. mangostana* and include, among others, α-, β-, and γ-mangostins [166, 167].

G. mangostana preparations are also used against diabetes in various traditional systems [161–163] including Surinamese Jamu [51]. Support for this use is provided by

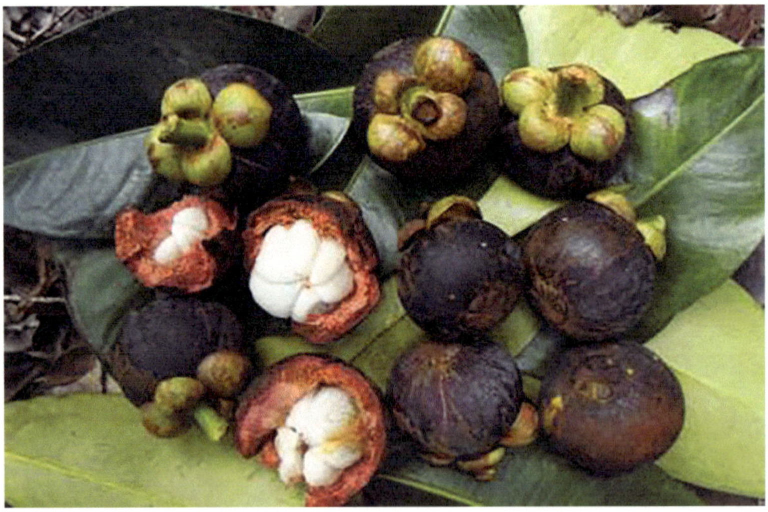

Figure 7.
Fruits of the mangosteen Garcinia mangostana *L. (Clusiaceae) (from: https://images.app.goo.gl/6tU39NW2ABubRr7t7).*

the reduction in blood glucose levels and/or insulin resistance as well as the increase in insulin levels noted in high-fat diet and streptozotocin-induced type II diabetic and nephropathic rodents treated with pericarp extracts enriched with xanthones [168–170]. The *G. mangostana* preparations also improved, among others, oral glucose tolerance and the histology of the β-cells [168–170] as well as blood lipid profiles in the animal models [171, 172]. These effects have been ascribed to α-mangostin and γ-mangostin, which elicited comparable antidiabetic activities as the crude *G. mangostana* extracts *in vivo* [173], stimulated insulin secretion in cultured INS-1 rat insulinoma cells, and protected the cells from apoptotic damage [174], and decreased insulin resistance in primary cultures of newly differentiated human adipocytes [175].

The antidiabetic activities of *G. mangostana* have been associated with the antioxidant properties of the xanthones in the plant, which elicited potent DPPH free radical-scavenging activity, superoxide dismutase and catalase stimulatory activities, and notable malondialdehyde inhibitory activity [168–170]. Furthermore, the *G. mangostana* preparations inhibited α-amylase and α-glycosidase activities *in vitro* [176, 177], which was consistent with the lowering of postprandial blood glucose levels by an ethanol extract of the pericarp in streptozotocin-induced diabetic rats [177]. Candidates for the anti-enzymatic effects are the xanthone garcimangostin A which displayed acarbose-like α-amylase inhibitory activity in molecular docking studies [178], and oligomeric proanthocyanidins as well as α-mangostin and γ-mangostin that inhibited α-amylase and α-glucosidase *in vitro* [170, 176, 177].

Until today, there is only some indirect evidence on the clinical efficacy of *G. mangostana*. Thus, a fruit juice herbal blend, either alone or in combination with parts from other plants, and a fruit extract in a capsule formulation led to a reduction in body weight, body mass index, and waist circumference of non-diabetic obese patients [179–181]. Since these positive changes were accompanied by an improvement in insulin sensitivity [181], the data from these studies have merit.

8. Plants with hypoglycemic properties associated with Surinamese from Chinese origin

8.1 Araliaceae: *Panax notoginseng* (Burkill) F.H.Chen

The Chinese ginseng *Panax notoginseng* (Burkill) F.H.Chen (Araliaceae) (**Figure 8**) is probably native to south-eastern China and Vietnam but has spread to forests from China to the Himalayas and Myanmar. *P. notoginseng* must not be confused with other *Panax* species such as the Asian ginseng *P. ginseng* C.A. Meyer and the American ginseng *P. quinquefolius* L., which it superficially resembles. However, an important distinguishing characteristic of *P. notoginseng* is the presence of three petioles with seven leaflets each. This is the reason this plant is referred to in China as "sān-qī," meaning "the three-seven herb." *P. notoginseng* is either cultivated or gathered from the wild, and the interest in this plant is particularly for its root and rhizome which are used to prepare foods, health products, beauty products, dietary supplements, and medicines [182].

P. notoginseng dried root and rhizome are very common ingredients of traditional Chinese medicines including those used by Surinamese-Chinese [183]. A few indications are arteriosclerosis, high blood pressure, coronary heart disease, and angina pectoris; internal and external bleedings ranging from nosebleeds to intracerebral hemorrhages; inflammatory conditions such as osteoarthritis and rheumatoid

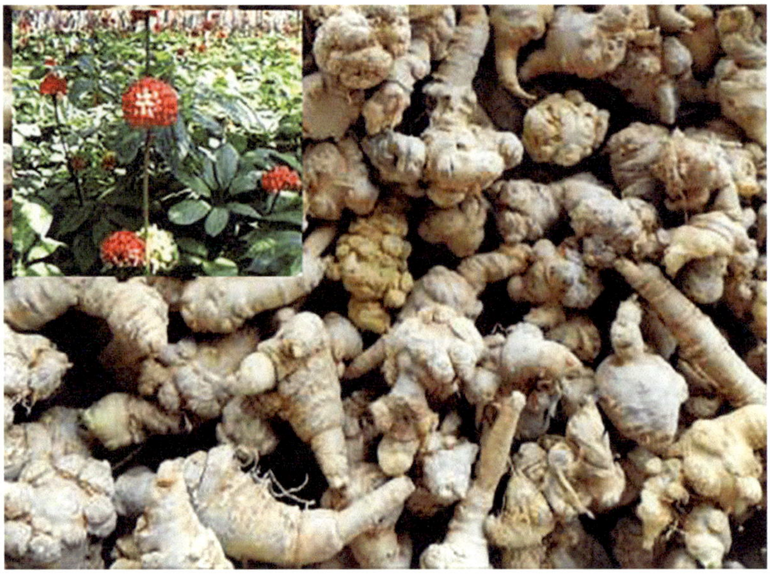

Figure 8.
Rhizmes of the Chinese ginseng or sān-qī Panax notoginseng (Burkill) F.H.Chen (Araliaceae) (from: https://images.app.goo.gl/NB2rRHGPbEQrg1id9). In de insert de flower of the plant (from: https://images.app.goo.gl/HbVFx8SkBDNy2zp37).

arthritis; pains and swellings; liver disease; poor cognitive ability or mood; and substandard athletic performance and muscle soreness following exercise [184, 185]. Pharmacological studies supported some of these uses, showing, among others, beneficial effects on the cardiovascular system and cerebrovascular diseases; hemostatic, wound healing, and angiogenesis-modulating effects; anti-inflammatory, antioxidant, antimicrobial, and antiviral activities; estrogen-like properties; cognitive enhancing, antidepressant, and anxiolytic activities; as well as performance-enhancing activities [185–187].

The main active constituents believed to be responsible for these activities are the unique triterpene saponins in the plant called dammarane saponines, which consist of a dammarane skeleton (17 carbons in a four-ring structure) with various sugar moieties attached to the C-3 and C-20 positions [185–187]. The biologically most important dammarane saponines in *P. notoginseng* are believed to be the notoginsenosides [185–187]. This was the rationale for developing and patenting a saponin-enriched *P. notoginseng* product as a traditional treatment for cardiovascular disorders in China [188]. Other phytochemicals in *P. notoginseng* with pharmacological activity are polysaccharides such as starch-like glucans and pectin; amino acids and proteins; volatile oils comprising, among others, sesquiterpenoids; polyacetylenes, phytosterols, and flavonoids, as well as the triacylglycerol trilinolein [186].

P. notoginseng root and rhizome extracts as well as purified notoginsenosides or notoginsenoside-containing formulations have also been used for thousands of years in traditional Chinese medicine for treating the symptoms of diabetes [182]. The results from many pharmacological studies—both *in vivo* and *in vitro*—have supported this use [189, 190]. For instance, the administration of *P. notoginseng* saponins led to a decrease in blood glucose in alloxan-induced diabetic mice [191], hyperglycemic and obese KK-Ay mice [192, 193], and high-fat diet-induced diabetic KKAy mice [194]. These effects were accompanied by an increased synthesis of liver glycogen in normal mice [191] and improved serum insulin levels, glucose tolerance, insulin resistance, glomerular lesions [192], and body weight in diabetic animals [192–195]. The latter observation was consistent with the *in vitro* and *in vivo* anti-obesity effects of notoginsenosides [195].

These findings were in accordance with the increased (insulin-stimulated) glucose uptake by a rat liver homogenate [191], 3 T3-L1 murine adipocyte-like cells [196], and cultured C2C12 skeletal myoblast [197] following exposure to *P. notogensing* saponins, as well as the concomitant increase in the expression of several elements of signaling pathways considered important in the pathogenesis of diabetes including the glucose transporter type 4 GLUT4, p-PI3K, and p-Akt [194, 196]. *P. notoginseng* saponins treatment also increased intracellular superoxide dismutase and catalase levels and decreased reactive oxygen species and malondialdehyde content in rat retinal capillary endothelial cells exposed to high glucose [198]. All these data taken together suggest that *P. notoginseng* and its notoginsenosides affect multiple metabolic pathways involved in glucose homeostasis, including, among others, glucose absorption, glucose transport, and/or glucose disposal, as well as insulin secretion and binding.

A few clinical studies support the antidiabetic efficacy of *P. notoginseng* in diabetic patients. For instance, the daily intake of 3 g of *P. notoginseng* for 3 days lowered postprandial glycemia in untrained non-diabetic adults of 20–45 years when compared to one cycling exercise of 30 min on day 3 prior to the glucose intake by these men [199]. Furthermore, the saponins delayed the progress of diabetic nephropathy [200] and elicited beneficial effects in type 2 diabetic angiopathy [201]. And a meta-analysis suggested that some commercial products containing *P. notoginseng* saponins may well be beneficial as adjuvant therapy for diabetic kidney disease [200].

8.2. Lauraceae: *Cinnamomum cassia* (L.) J.Presl

Cinnamomum cassia (L.) J.Presl (Lauraceae) (**Figure 9**), also called Chinese cassia, Chinese cinnamon, or "guān guì" in Mandarin (referring to something precious or valuable), is an evergreen tree that originates from southern China and has spread to various neighboring countries in southern and south-eastern Asia. *C. cassia* is, along with several other *Cinnamomum* species including the Ceylon cinnamon *C. verum*, the Saigon cinnamon *C. loureiroi*, the Indonesian cinnamon *C. burmannii*, and the Malabar cinnamon *C. citriodorum* (from the Malabar region in India), widely cultivated for its aromatic, reddish inner bark that gives the spice cinnamon after drying. Cinnamon is used as a flavoring agent for confectionery, desserts, pastries, and meat dishes including many savory curry recipes. One of the several flavoring substances is coumarin, a benzopyrone that has, however, anticoagulant properties and can cause liver damage in sensitive individuals if consumed in larger amounts [202].

C. cassia has a long traditional use for treating a wide variety of diseases, particularly in China [203–205] but also in the Chinese community in Suriname. Preparations from mainly the bark of this plant are used against, among others, microbial and parasitic infections; the common cold; inflammation; joint pain and hernia; loss of appetite stomach, spasms, nausea and vomiting, flatulence, and diarrhea; chest pain; kidney disorders; bed-wetting; erectile dysfunction; menopausal symptoms, menstrual problems, and to cause abortions; as well as hypertension, cancer, and diabetes [203–205]. Some of these traditional uses are supported by the many pharmacological studies carried out with *C. cassia* preparations, cinnamon spice, and isolated compounds from the plant showing antimicrobial, antiviral, antioxidant,

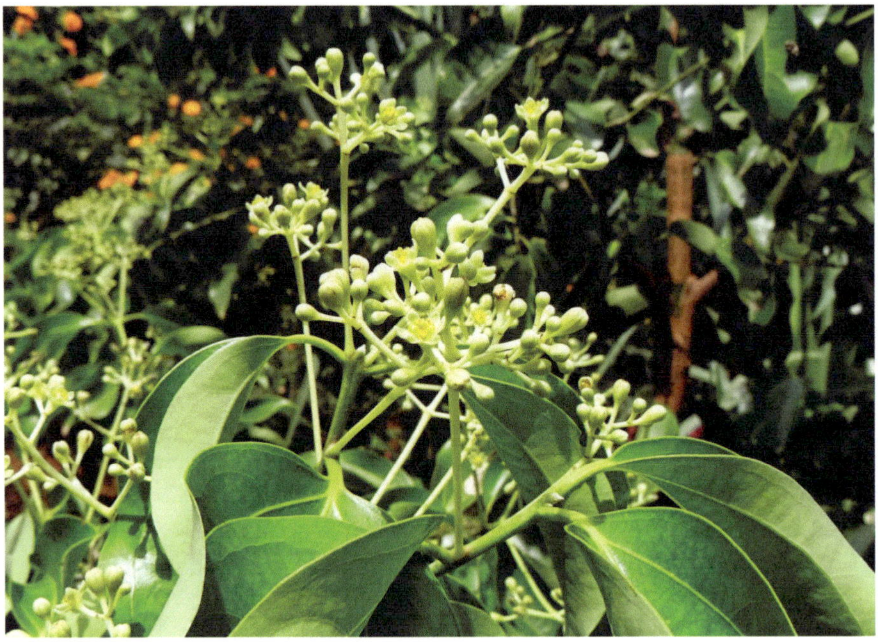

Figure 9.
Leaves, flowers, and fruits of the Chinese cassia or guān guì Cinnamomum cassia *(L.) J.Presl (Lauraceae) (from: https://images.app.goo.gl/HGEBbvErrXoR43UL9).*

anti-inflammatory, gastroprotective, nematicidal, acaricidal, repellent, anti-obesity, anti-angiogenic, and anticancer activities [203–205]. Phytochemical analyses have shown the presence in the plant of bioactive phenylpropanoids including cinnamaldehyde that is considered its main pharmacologically active ingredient (and that also contributes to its flavor and aroma), as well as terpenoids, glycosides, lignans, and lactones in addition to coumarin [203–205].

There is also ample preclinical evidence for hypoglycemic activity of *C. cassia*. For instance, aqueous extracts of the bark decreased blood glucose concentration in streptozotocin-induced diabetic mice [206, 207], type II diabetic C57BIKsj db/db mice [208, 209], and rats challenged by a glucose load [210]. The *C. cassia* preparations were also able to stimulate the release of insulin from the insulin-secreting rat cell line INS-1 *in vitro* [210] and to increase plasma insulin levels in the animal models [208, 210]. In addition, serum insulin levels and HDL-cholesterol levels were increased while those of triglycerides, total cholesterol, and LDL were decreased [208, 209].

The hypoglycemic effects of *C. cassia* were accompanied by a reduction in malondialdehye levels [206] and a rise in glutathione levels and glutathione peroxidase activity [211], suggesting the involvement of antioxidant activity in its mechanism of action. This is supported by the abundance of polyphenolic compounds with considerable antioxidant activity in the plant [204, 205, 212] and by the decrease of plasma malondialdehyde levels in overweight and obese adults with prediabetes who had consumed the *C. cassia* bark-based supplement Cinnulin PF® [213]. In addition, both *in vitro* and *in vivo* studies reported that cinnamon led to a decrease in α-amylase and α-glycosidase activities [208, 214–216]; an increase in hepatic glycogenesis [217], and an increase in the consumption of extracellular glucose in both insulin-resistant

HepG2 and normal HepG2 cells [207]. Thus, *C. cassia* may alleviate diabetes through its antioxidant activity, by delaying carbohydrate digestion and lowering postprandial glucose levels, by storing excess glucose in the liver, and by improving insulin resistance and sensitivity.

In some clinical studies, the consumption of cinnamon spice or a phenolic-enriched extract of *C. cassia* bark indeed led to a reduction in fasting [218, 219] and postprandial blood glucose levels [220–223] as well as an improvement in insulin sensitivity in healthy [220, 222–224], obese [223, 224], and type 2 diabetic patients [219]. Cinnamon and powdered aqueous *C. cassia* bark extract also caused a delay in gastric emptying [220], and enhanced insulin sensitivity [224], as well as improvements in fasting plasma glucose and HbA1c along with lipid profiles in type 2 diabetic patients [218]. However, other studies reported no effect of cinnamon spice or encapsulated *C. cassia* bark on blood sugar levels, insulin sensitivity, oral glucose tolerance, blood lipid profile, and/or liver enzymes in either normal-weight non-diabetic individuals or obese diabetic subjects [225–227].

9. Concluding remarks

Diabetes remains one of the most prevalent diseases of mankind. Despite the many therapeutic options available, this condition is often treated with a variety of traditional medicines in many parts of the world. This chapter has extensively addressed eight plants and plant-derived preparations with hypoglycemic properties, two of which are traditionally used against diabetes by each of the four largest ethnic groups in Suriname. *R. tuberosa* and *G. globosa* are associated with the Afro-Surinamese, *S. cumini* and *A. marmelos* with the Surinamese Hindustani, *S. crispa* and *G. mangostana* with the Surinamese Javanese, and *P. notoginseng* and *C. cassia* with the Surinamese Chinese. As mentioned above, the prevalence of diabetes and other non-communicable diseases is relatively high in Suriname [35–39], while most Surinamese have largely remained true to their cultural customs [28].

However, as summarized in **Table 2**, despite the availability of many preclinical observations on antidiabetic/hypoglycemic activity of preparations from the plants, the scientific evidence to back up these data is disappointingly meager. Notably, four of the eight plants (*R. tuberosa*, *G. globosa*, *S. crispa*, and *G. mangostana*) had not even undergone clinical testing, while the clinical findings of the remaining four (*S. cumini*, *A. marmelos*, *P. notoginseng*, and *C. cassia*) were in general inconsistent, some reporting positive effects in diabetic patients, others mentioning negative effects. On the bright side, there were in all cases suggestions about the pharmacologically active ingredients and mechanisms that may be involved in the putative antidiabetic/hypoglycemic activities of the plants (**Table 2**). Then again, it remains to be seen whether these findings also apply in the clinic.

These data clearly indicate the shortcomings of the scientific evidence accumulated so far to support the use of these plants against diabetes. This raises not only the possibility that patients treat their disease with substances that may be ineffective, but also that they may run the risk of unknown or unforeseen adverse effects or interactions with allopathic medicines or food constituents. For these reasons, it is necessary to subject these plants to systematic and large-scale clinical trials to definitely establish their roles in the treatment of diabetes. Obviously, these studies must be carried out with standardized preparations and uniform doses and administration schedules. The results from these studies are particularly important to countries such as Suriname, where a large proportion of the population relies on traditional herbal medicinal products.

Author details

Dennis R.A. Mans
Faculty of Medical Sciences, Department of Pharmacology, Anton de Kom University of Suriname, Paramaribo, Suriname

*Address all correspondence to: dennismans16@gmail.com;
dennis_mans@yahoo.com

References

[1] Petersmann A, Müller-Wieland D, Müller UA, Landgraf R, Nauck M, Freckmann G, et al. Definition, classification and diagnosis of diabetes mellitus. Experimental and Clinical Endocrinology and Diabetes. 2019;**127**:S1-S7. DOI: 10.1055/a-1018-9078

[2] Cloete L. Diabetes mellitus: An overview of the types, symptoms, complications and management. Nursing Standard. 2022;**37**:61-66. DOI: 10.7748/ns.2021.e11709

[3] International Diabetes Federation. IDF Diabetes Atlas 10th edition, 2021. Suriname. Diabetes report 2000-2045. Available from: https://diabetesatlas.org/data/en/country/190/sr.html [Accessed March 21, 2022]

[4] Ohiagu F, Chikezie P, Chikezie C. Pathophysiology of diabetes mellitus complications: Metabolic events and control. Biomedical Research and Therapy. 2021;**8**:4243-4257. DOI: 10.15419/bmrat.v8i3.663

[5] World Health Organization. The Top 10 Causes of Death. 2020. Available from: https://www.who.int/news-room/fact-sheets/detail/the-top-10-causes-of-death. [Accessed March 21, 2022]

[6] Huang Y, Karuranga S, Boyko EJ, Malanda B. Diabetes prevalence in North America and Caribbean region in 2017 and 2045. Diabetes. 2018;**67**:1676. DOI: 10.2337/db18-1676-P

[7] Boyne M. Diabetes in the Caribbean: Trouble in paradise. Insulin. 2009;**4**:94-105. DOI: 10.1016/S1557-0843(09)80018-3

[8] American Diabetes Association. Professional practice committee: Standards of medical care in diabetes—2022. Diabetes Care. 2022;**45**:S3. DOI: 10.2337/dc22-SPPC

[9] World Health Organization. Classification of Diabetes Mellitus. Geneva: World Health Organization; 2019. Licence: CC BY-NC-SA 3.0 IGO

[10] Beulens J, Rutters F, Rydén L, Schnell O, Mellbin L, Hart HE, et al. Risk and management of pre-diabetes. European Journal of Preventive Cardiology. 2019;**26**:47-54. DOI: 10.1177/2047487319880041

[11] Kahanovitz L, Sluss PM, Russell SJ. Type 1 diabetes—A clinical perspective. Point Care. 2017;**16**:37-40. DOI: 10.1097/POC.0000000000000125

[12] Reed J, Bain S, Kanamarlapudi V. A review of current trends with type 2 diabetes epidemiology, aetiology, pathogenesis, treatments and future perspectives. Diabetes, Metabolic Syndrome and Obesity. 2021;**14**:3567-3602. DOI: 10.2147/DMSO.S319895

[13] McIntyre HD, Catalano P, Zhang C, Desoye G, Mathiesen ER, Damm P. Gestational diabetes mellitus. Nature Reviews. Disease Primers. 2019;**5**:47. DOI: 10.1038/s41572-019-0098-8

[14] Lemelman MB, Letourneau L, Greeley SAW. Neonatal diabetes mellitus: An update on diagnosis and management. Clinics in Perinatology. 2018;**45**:41-59. DOI: 10.1016/j.clp.2017.10.006

[15] Skoczek D, Dulak J, Kachamakova-Trojanowska N. Maturity onset diabetes of the young—New approaches for disease modelling. International Journal of Molecular

Sciences. 2021;**22**:7553. DOI: 10.3390/ijms22147553

[16] Rosanio FM, Di Candia F, Occhiati L, Fedi L, Malvone FP, Foschini DF, et al. Wolfram syndrome type 2: A systematic review of a not easily identifiable clinical spectrum. International Journal of Environmental Research and Public Health. 2022;**19**:835. DOI: 10.3390/ijerph19020835

[17] Kelsey R, Manderson Koivula FN, McClenaghan NH, Kelly C. Cystic fibrosis-related diabetes: Pathophysiology and therapeutic challenges. Clinical Medicine Insights: Endocrinology and Diabetes. 2019;**12**:1179551419851770. DOI: 10.1177/1179551419851770

[18] Trivedi CD, Pitchumoni CS. Drug-induced pancreatitis: An update. Journal of Clinical Gastroenterology. 2005;**39**:709-716. DOI: 10.1097/01.mcg.0000173929.60115.b4

[19] Hirsch IB, Gaudiani LM. A new look at brittle diabetes. Journal of Diabetes and its Complications. 2021;**35**:107646. DOI: 10.1016/j.jdiacomp.2020.107646

[20] Pivonello R, De Leo M, Vitale P, Cozzolino A, Simeoli C, De Martino MC, et al. Pathophysiology of diabetes mellitus in Cushing's syndrome. Neuroendocrinology. 2010;**92**:77-81. DOI: 10.1159/000314319

[21] Karamanou M, Protogerou A, Tsoucalas G, Androutsos G, Poulakou-Rebelakou E. Milestones in the history of diabetes mellitus: The main contributors. World Journal of Diabetes. 2016;7:1-7. DOI: 10.4239/wjd.v7.i1.1

[22] Kesavadev J, Saboo B, Krishna MB, Krishnan G. Evolution of insulin delivery devices: From syringes, pens, and pumps to DIY artificial pancreas. Diabetes Therapy. 2020;**11**:1251-1269. DOI: 10.1007/s13300-020-00831-z

[23] Hirsch IB, Juneja R, Beals JM, Antalis CJ, Wright EE. The evolution of insulin and how it informs therapy and treatment choices. Endocrine Reviews. 2020;**41**:733-755. DOI: 10.1210/endrev/bnaa015

[24] Cernea S, Raz I. Insulin therapy: Future perspectives. American Journal of Therapeutics. 2020;**27**:e121-e132. DOI: 10.1097/MJT.0000000000001076

[25] Padhi S, Nayak AK, Behera A. Type II diabetes mellitus: A review on recent drug based therapeutics. Biomedicine and Pharmacotherapy. 2020;**131**:110708. DOI: 10.1016/j.biopha.2020.110708

[26] Dahlén AD, Dashi G, Maslov I, Attwood MM, Jonsson J, Trukhan V, et al. Trends in antidiabetic drug discovery: FDA approved drugs, new drugs in clinical trials and global sales. Frontiers in Pharmacology. 2022;**12**:807548. DOI: 10.3389/fphar.2021.807548

[27] Algemeen Bureau voor de Statistiek/Censuskantoor. Suriname in cijfers 2013/05. Resultaten achtste (8ste) volks- en woningtelling in Suriname (volume 1) (General Bureau of Statistics/Census office. Suriname in numbers 2013/05. Results of the Eight General Census of Suriname). Demografische en sociale karakteristieken en migratie (Demographic and social characteristics and migration). Paramaribo: Algemeen Bureau voor de Statistiek; 2013

[28] Mans DRA, Ganga D, Kartopawiro J. Meeting of the minds: Traditional herbal medicine in multiethnic Suriname (chapter 6). In: El-Shemy H, editor. Aromatic and Medicinal Plants—Back to Nature. Rijeka: InTech; 2017. pp. 111-132. DOI: 10.5772/66509

[29] Hammond DS. Forest conservation and management in the Guiana shield (chapter 1). In: Hammond DS, editor. Tropical Rainforests of the Guiana Shield. Wallingford: CABI Publishing; 2005. pp. 1-14

[30] Algemeen Bureau voor de Statistiek. Suriname in cijfers 303-2014-04 (General Bureau of Statistics. Suriname in numbers 303-2014-04). Basis indicatoren (Basic indicators). Paramaribo: Algemeen Bureau voor de Statistiek; 2014

[31] The World Bank Group. Data— Suriname [Internet]. Washington, DC, USA: World Bank Group; 2021. Available from: https://data.worldbank.org/country/suriname?view=chart [Accessed: March 11, 2022]

[32] Budreviciute A, Damiati S, Sabir DK, Onder K, Schuller-Goetzburg P, Plakys G, et al. Management and prevention strategies for non-communicable diseases (NCDs) and their risk factors. Frontiers in Public Health. 2020;**8**:574111. DOI: 10.3389/fpubh.2020.574111

[33] Baldew SS, Krishnadath IS, Smits CC, Toelsie JR, Vanhees L, Cornelissen V. Self-reported physical activity behavior of a multi-ethnic adult population within the urban and rural setting in Suriname. BMC Public Health. 2015;**15**:485. DOI: 10.1186/s12889-015-1807-1

[34] Suriname Ministry of Health. Global School-Based Student Health Survey. Paramaribo: Suriname Ministry of Health; 2009

[35] World Health Organization. Noncommunicable Diseases (NCD) Country Profiles. Suriname. Geneva: World Health Organization; 2014

[36] Krishnadath ISK, Toelsie JR, Hofman A, Jaddoe VWV. Ethnic disparities in the prevalence of metabolic syndrome and its risk factors in the Suriname Health Study: A cross-sectional population study. BMJ Open. 2016;**6**:e013183. DOI: 10.1136/bmjopen-2016-013183

[37] Punwasi W. Doodsoorzaken in Suriname 2010-2011 (Causes of Death in Suriname 2010-2011). Paramaribo: Bureau for Public Health (Ministry of Health); 2012

[38] Krishnadath IS, Smits CC, Jaddoe VW, Hofman A, Toelsie JR. A national surveillance survey on noncommunicable disease risk factors: Suriname Health Study Protocol. JMIR Research Protocols. 2015;**4**:e75. DOI: 10.2196/resprot.4205

[39] Krishnadath ISK, Nahar-van Venrooij LM, Jaddoe VWV, Toelsie JR. Ethnic differences in prediabetes and diabetes in the Suriname Health Study. BMJ Open Diabetes Research and Care. 2016;**4**:e000186. DOI: 10.1136/bmjdrc-2015-000186

[40] De Medeiros PM, Soldati GT, Alencar NL, Vandebroek I, Pieroni A, Hanazaki N, et al. The use of medicinal plants by migrant people: Adaptation, maintenance, and replacement. Evidence-Based Complementary and Alternative Medicine. 2012;**2012**:807452. DOI: 10.1155/2012/807452

[41] Grennes T. The Columbian exchange and the reversal of fortune. Cato Journal. 2007;**27**:91-107

[42] Nunn N, Qian N. The Columbian exchange: A history of disease, food, and ideas. Journal of Economic Perspectives. 2010;**24**:163-188. DOI: 10.1257/jep.24.2.163

[43] Crosby AW. The Columbian Exchange: Biological and Cultural

Consequences of 1492. Westport (CT): Greenwood Press; 1972

[44] Singh P, Chauhan V, Tiwari BK, Chauhan SS, Simon S, Bilal S, et al. An overview on okra (*Abelmoschus esculentus*) and its importance as a nutritive vegetable in the world. International Journal of Pharmacy and Biological Sciences. 2014;**4**:227-233

[45] Alpern SB. Exotic plants of western Africa: Where they came from and when. History in Africa. 2008;**35**:63-102

[46] Carney JA, Rosomoff RN. In the Shadow of Slavery: Africa's Botanical Legacy in the Atlantic World. Berkeley (CA): University of California Press; 2009

[47] Diallo BO, Joly HI, McKey D, Hosaert-McKey M, Chevallier MH. Genetic diversity of *Tamarindus indica* populations: Any clues on the origin from its current distribution? African Journal of Biotechnology. 2007;**6**:853-860

[48] Vilar Dde A, Vilar MS, de Lima e Moura TF, Raffin FN, de Oliveira MR, Franco CF, et al. Traditional uses, chemical constituents, and biological activities of *Bixa orellana* L.: A review. ScientificWorld Journal. 2014;**2014**:857292. DOI: 10.1155/2014/857292

[49] Gómez-Betancur I, Benjumea D. Traditional use of the genus *Renealmia* and *Renealmia alpinia* (Rottb.) Maas (Zingiberaceae): A review in the treatment of snakebites. Asian Pacific Journal of Tropical Medicine. 2014;**7**:S574-S582

[50] Van Andel T, Maas P, Dobreff J. Ethnobotanical notes from Daniel Rolander's *Diarium Surinamicum* (1754-1756): Are these plants still used in Suriname today? Taxon. 2012;**61**:852-863

[51] Tjong Ayong G. Het gebruik van medicinale planten door de Javaanse bevolkingsgroep in Suriname (The Use of Medicinal Plants by the Javanese in Suriname). Instituut voor de Opleiding van Leraren: Paramaribo; 1989

[52] Sedoc NO. Afrosurinaamse natuurgeneeswijzen: Bevattende meer dan tweehonderd meest gebruikelijke geneeskrachtige kruiden (Afro-Surinamese natural remedies: Over two hundred commonly used medicinal herbs). Paramaribo: Vaco Press; 1992

[53] Raghoenandan UPD. Etnobotanisch onderzoek bij de Hindoestaanse bevolkingsgroep in Suriname (An ethnobotanical investigation among Hindustanis in Suriname) [thesis]. Paramaribo: Anton de Kom Universiteit van Suriname; 1994

[54] DeFilipps RA, Maina SL, Crepin J. Medicinal Plants of the Guianas (Guyana, Surinam, French Guiana). Washington, DC: Smithsonian Institution; 2004

[55] Van Andel TR, Ruysschaert S. Medicinale en Rituele Planten van Suriname (Medicinal and Ritual Plants of Suriname). Amsterdam: KIT Publishers; 2011

[56] Chothani DL, Patel MB, Vaghasiya HU, Mishira SH. Review on *Ruellia tuberosa* (cracker plant). Pharmacognosy Journal. 2010;**2**:506-512

[57] Afzal K, Uzair M, Chaudhary BA, Ahmad A, Afzal S, Saadullah M. Genus *Ruellia*: Pharmacological and phytochemical importance in ethnopharmacology. Acta Poloniae Pharmaceutica. 2015;**72**:821-827

[58] Samy MN, Sugimoto S, Matsunami K, Otsuka H, Kamel MS. Chemical constituents and biological

activities of genus *Ruellia*. International Journal of Pharmacognosy. 2015;**2**:270-279. DOI: 10.1007/s10600-013-0549-5

[59] Shahwar D, Ullah S, Ahmad M, Ullah S, Ahmad N, Khan MA. Hypoglycemic activity of *Ruellia tuberosa* Linn (Acanthaceae) in normal and alloxan-induced diabetic rabbits. Iranian Journal of Pharmaceutical Sciences. 2011;7:107-115

[60] Rajan M, Kumar VK, Kumar PS, Swathi KR, Haritha S. Antidiabetic, antihyperlipidaemic and hepatoprotective activity of methanolic extract of *Ruellia tuberosa* Linn leaves in normal and alloxan induced diabetic rats. Journal of Chemical and Pharmaceutical Research. 2012;**4**:2860-2868

[61] Wulan DR, Utomo EP, Mahdi C. Antidiabetic activity of *Ruellia tuberosa* L., role of α-amylase inhibitor: *In silico*, *in vitro*, and *in vivo* approaches. Biochemistry Research International. 2015;**2015**:349261. DOI: 10.1155/2015/349261

[62] Chang W-C, Huang D-W, Chenc J-A, Chang Y-F, Wu JS-B, Shen S-C. Protective effect of *Ruellia tuberosa* L. extracts against abnormal expression of hepatic detoxification enzymes in diabetic rats. RSC Advances. 2018;**8**:21596-21605. DOI: 10.1039/C8RA03321H

[63] Ko C-Y, Lin R-H, Zeng Y-M, Chang W-C, Huang D-W, Wu JS-B, et al. Ameliorative effect of *Ruellia tuberosa* L. on hyperglycemia in type 2 diabetes mellitus and glucose uptake in mouse C2C12 myoblasts. Food Science and Nutrition. 2018;**6**:2414-2422. DOI: 10.1002/fsn3.840

[64] Roosdiana A, Permata FS, Fitriani RI, Umam K, Safitri A. *Ruellia tuberosa* L. extract improves histopathology and lowers malondialdehyde levels and TNF alpha expression in the kidney of streptozotocin-induced diabetic rats. Veterinary Medicine International. 2020;**2020**:8812758. DOI: 10.1155/2020/8812758

[65] Safitri A, Tirto Sari DR, Refsilangi B, Roosdiana A, Fatchiyah F. Histopathological profiles of rats (*Rattus norvegicus*) induced with streptozotocin and treated with aqueous root extracts of *Ruellia tuberosa* L. Veterinary Medicine International. 2021;**2021**:6938433. DOI: 10.1155/2021/6938433

[66] Chaitanya BK, Babu SR, Ramesh C, Ravella A, Vardhan J, Atigari DV. Hypolipidemic and anti-oxidant activity of *Ruellia tuberosa* Linn. International Journal of Pharmacy and Biological Sciences. 2012;**2**:63-72

[67] Lin C-F, Huang Y-L, Cheng L-Y, Sheu S-J, Chen C-C. Bioactive flavonoids from *Ruellia tuberosa*. Journal of Chinese Medicine. 2006;**17**:103-109

[68] Dos Santos JM, Tewari S, Mendes RH. The role of oxidative stress in the development of diabetes mellitus and its complications. Journal of Diabetes Research. 2019;**2019**:4189813. DOI: 10.1155/2019/4189813

[69] Singh A, Kukreti R, Saso L, Kukreti S. Mechanistic insight into oxidative stress-triggered signaling pathways and type 2 diabetes. Molecules. 2022;**27**:950. DOI: 10.3390/molecules27030950

[70] Ananthakrishnan M, Doss VA. Effect of 50% hydro-ethanolic leaf extracts of *Ruellia tuberosa* L. and *Dipteracanthus patulus* (Jacq.) on lipid profile in alloxan induced diabetic rats. International Journal of Preventive Medicine. 2013;**4**:744-747

[71] Trinh PTN, An PN, Tuan NT, Thuy NTL, Danh TT, Dung LT. Research

on phytochemical and alfa-glucosidase inhibitory activity of ethyl acetate fraction of *Ruellia tuberosa*. Vietnam Journal of Science and Technology. 2018;**56**:106-112

[72] Tundis R, Loizzo MR, Menichini F. Natural products as alpha-amylase and alpha-glucosidase inhibitors and their hypoglycaemic potential in the treatment of diabetes: An update. Mini-Reviews in Medicinal Chemistry. 2010;**10**:315-331. DOI: 10.2174/138955710791331007

[73] Xu JH, Lo YM, Chang WC, Huang DW, Wu JS, Jhang YY, et al. Identification of bioactive components from *Ruellia tuberosa* L. on improving glucose uptake in TNF-α-induced insulin-resistant mouse FL83B hepatocytes. Evidence-Based Complementary and Alternative Medicine. 2020;**2020**:6644253. DOI: 10.1155/2020/6644253

[74] Roriz CL, Barros L, Prieto MA, Morales P, Ferreira ICFR. Floral parts of *Gomphrena globosa* L. as a novel alternative source of betacyanins: Optimization of the extraction using response surface methodology. Food Chemistry. 2017;**229**:223-234. DOI: 10.1016/j.foodchem.2017.02.073

[75] Kumorkiewicz-Jamro A, Świergosz T, Sutor K, Spórna-Kucab A, Wybraniec S. Multi-colored shades of betalains: Recent advances in betacyanin chemistry. Natural Product Reports. 2021;**38**:2315-2346. DOI: 10.1039/D1NP00018G

[76] Ilyas M, Tarnam A, Begum N. Biological potential and phytopharmacological screening of *Gomphrena* species. Global Journal of Pharmacology. 2013;7:457-464

[77] Esmat AU, Mittapally S. A review on *Gomphrena globosa* (L.). International Journal of Research in Ayurveda and Pharmacy. 2020;**11**:78-84. DOI: 10.7897/2277-4343.110366

[78] Silva LR, Valentão P, Faria J, Ferreres F, Sousa C, Gil-Izquierdo A, et al. Phytochemical investigations and biological potential screening with cellular and non-cellular models of globe amaranth (*Gomphrena globosa* L.) inflorescences. Food Chemistry. 2012;**135**:756-763. DOI: 10.1016/j.foodchem.2012.05.015

[79] Hamiduzzaman M. Significant hypoglycemic activity from *Gomphrena globosa* (Amaranthaceae) in mice model. Universal Journal of Pharmacy. 2013;**2**:68-72

[80] Omodamiro OD, Jimoh MA. Hypoglycemic effect of ethanolic leaves extracts of Anacardium occidentalis and *Gomphrena globosa* plants on alloxan induced-diabetic rats. Journal of Chemical and Pharmaceutical Research. 2014;**6**:492-498

[81] Sherif ATY. *In vitro* antidiabetic, antioxidant and antiglycation activity of ethanolic leaf extract of *Gomphrena globosa* (Linn.). Asian Journal of Biological and Life Sciences. 2021;**10**:101-109. DOI: 10.5530/ajbls.2021.10.16

[82] Ningrum NA, Wijayanti N. Antioxidant properties of *Gomphrena globosa* leaves extract. AIP Conference Proceedings. 2020;**2260**:040022. DOI: 10.1063/5.0015689

[83] Ayyanar M, Subash-Babu P. *Syzygium cumini* (L.) Skeels: A review of its phytochemical constituents and traditional uses. Asian Pacific Journal of Tropical Biomedicine. 2012;**2**:240-246. DOI: 10.1016/S2221-1691(12)60050-1

[84] Sharma R, Oberoi K, Sharma K, Nagraik R, Kumar D, Sharma A, et al. Bioactive compounds and ethnomedicinal

uses of *Syzygium cumini* (L.) Skeels—A comprehensive review. Annals of the university Dunarea de Jos of Galati. Fascicle VI—Food Technology. 2020;**44**:230-254. DOI: 10.35219/foodtechnology.2020.1.14

[85] Srivastava S, Chandra D. Pharmacological potentials of *Syzygium cumini*: A review. Journal of the Science of Food and Agriculture. 2013;**93**:2084-2093. DOI: 10.1002/jsfa.6111

[86] Anjali V, Sindhu G, Girish C. A review on pharmacology and phytochemistry of *Syzygium cumini*. Indian Journal of Pharmaceutical and Biological Research. 2017;**5**:24-28

[87] Sharma SB, Nasir A, Prabhu KM, Murthy PS, Dev G. Hypoglycaemic and hypolipidemic effect of ethanolic extract of seeds of *Eugenia jambolana* in alloxan-induced diabetic rabbits. Journal of Ethnopharmacology. 2003;**85**:201-206. DOI: 10.1016/s0378-8741(02)00366-5

[88] Sridhar SB, Sheetal UD, Pai MRSM, Shastri MS. Preclinical evaluation of the antidiabetic effect of *Eugenia jambolana* seed powder in streptozotocin-diabetic rats. Brazilian Journal of Medical and Biological Research. 2005;**38**:463-468

[89] Yadav D, Lalit A, Singh S, Galgut JM, Beg MA. Evaluation of antidiabetic and phytochemical activity of 50% methanolic extract of jamun seed (*Syzygium cumini*). Search and Reserch. 2013;**4**:13-16

[90] Siddiqui MS, Sharma B, Ram G. Anti-hyperglycemic and anti-hyperlipemia effects of *Syzygium cumini* seed in alloxan induced diabetes mellitus in Swiss albino mice (Mus musculus). Medicinal and Aromatic Plants. 2014;**3**:166. DOI: 10.4172/2167-0412.1000166

[91] Ravi K, Rajasekaran S, Subramanian S. Antihyperlipidemic effect of *Eugenia jambolana* seed kernel on streptozotocin-induced diabetes in rats. Food and Chemical Toxicology. 2005;**43**:1433-1439. DOI: 10.1016/j.fct.2005.04.004

[92] Chattu M. Evaluation of antidiabetic activity for ethanolic extract of *Syzygium cumini* leaf in dexamethasone induced diabetic rats. Research in Pharmacy and Health Sciences. 2016;**2**:85-90. DOI: 10.32463/rphs.2016.v02i02.15

[93] Singh N, Gupta M. Effects of ethanolic extract of *Syzygium cumini* (Linn) seed powder on pancreatic islets of alloxan diabetic rats. Indian Journal of Experimental Biology. 2007;**45**:861-867

[94] Dusane MB, Joshi BN. Seeds of *Syzygium cumini* (L.) Skeels: Potential for islet regeneration in experimental diabetes. Zhong Xi Yi Jie He Xue Bao. 2011;**9**:1380-1387

[95] Sharma AK, Bharti S, Kumar R, Krishnamurthy B, Bhatia J, Kumari S, et al. *Syzygium cumini* ameliorates insulin resistance and β-cell dysfunction via modulation of PPAR, dyslipidemia, oxidative stress, and TNF-α in type 2 diabetic rats. Journal of Pharmacological Sciences. 2012;**119**:205-213. DOI: 10.1254/jphs.11184fp

[96] Rekha N, Balaji R, Deecaraman M. Antihyperglycemic and antihyper-lipidemic effects of extracts of the pulp of *Syzygium cumini* and bark of *Cinnamon zeylanicum* in streptozotocin-induced diabetic rats. Journal of Applied Biosciences. 2010;**28**:1718-1730

[97] Sharma SB, Nasir A, Prabhu KM, Murthy PS. Antihyperglycemic effect of the fruit-pulp of *Eugenia jambolana* in experimental diabetes mellitus. Journal of Ethnopharmacology.

2006;**104**:367-373. DOI: 10.1016/j.jep.2005.10.033

[98] Ravi K, Ramachandran B, Subramanian S. Protective effect of *Eugenia jambolana* seed kernel on tissue antioxidants in streptozotocin-induced diabetic rats. Biological and Pharmaceutical Bulletin. 2004;**27**:1212-1217. DOI: 10.1248/bpb.27.1212

[99] Ravi K, Ramachandran B, Subramanian S. Effect of *Eugenia jambolana* seed kernel on antioxidant defense system in streptozotocin-induced diabetes in rats. Life Sciences. 2004;**75**:2717-2731. DOI: 10.1016/j.lfs.2004.08.005

[100] Prince PS, Menon VP, Pari L. Hypoglycaemic activity of *Syzigium cumini* seeds: Effect on lipid peroxidation in alloxan diabetic rats. Journal of Ethnopharmacology. 1998;**61**:1-7. DOI: 10.1016/s0378-8741(98)00002-6

[101] Gajera HP, Gevariya SN, Hirpara DG, Patel SV, Golakiya BA. Antidiabetic and antioxidant functionality associated with phenolic constituents from fruit parts of indigenous black jamun (*Syzygium cumini* L.) landraces. Journal of Food Science and Technology. 2017;**54**:3180-3191. DOI: 10.1007/s13197-017-2756-8

[102] Mandal S, Barik B, Mallick C, De D, Ghosh D. Therapeutic effect of ferulic acid, an ethereal fraction of ethanolic extract of seed of *Syzygium cumini* against streptozotocin-induced diabetes in male rat. Methods and Findings in Experimental and Clinical Pharmacology. 2008;**30**:121-128

[103] Jung EH, Kim SR, Hwang IK, Ha TY. Hypoglycemic effects of a phenolic acid fraction of rice bran and ferulic acid in C57BL/KsJ-db/db mice. Journal of Agricultural and Food Chemistry. 2007;**55**:9800-9804. DOI: 10.1021/jf0714463

[104] KarthicK, KirthiramKS, SadasivamS, Thayumanavan B. Identification of α amylase inhibitors from *Syzygium cumini* Linn seeds. Indian Journal of Experimental Biology. 2008;**46**:677-680

[105] Shinde J, Taldone T, Barletta M, Kunaparaju N, Hu B, Kumar S, et al. Alpha-glucosidase inhibitory activity of *Syzygium cumini* (Linn.) Skeels seed kernel *in vitro* and in Goto-Kakizaki (GK) rats. Carbohydrate Research. 2008;**343**:1278-1281. DOI: 10.1016/j.carres.2008.03.003

[106] Syama HP, Arun KB, Sinumol G, Dhanya R, Anusree SS, Nisha P, et al. *Syzygium cumini* seed exhibits antidiabetic potential via multiple pathways involving inhibition of α-glucosidase, DPP-IV, glycation, and ameliorating glucose uptake in L6 cell lines. Journal of Food Processing and Preservation. 2018;**42**:e13464. DOI: 10.1111/jfpp.13464

[107] Helmstädter A. *Syzygium cumini* (L.) SKEELS (Myrtaceae) Against diabetes - 125 years of research. Die Pharmazie 2008;63:91-101

[108] Srivastava Y, Bhatt H, Gupta O, Gupta P. Hypoglycemia induced by *Syzygium cumini* Linn. seeds in diabetes mellitus. Asian Medical Journal. 1983;**26**:489-492

[109] Kohli K, Singh R. A clinical trial of jambu (*Eugenia jambolana*) in non-insulin dependant diabetes mellitus. Journal of Research in Ayurveda and Siddha. 1993;**13**:89-97

[110] Bopp A, De Bona KS, Bellé LP, Moresco RN, Moretto MB. *Syzygium cumini* inhibits adenosine deaminase activity and reduces

glucose levels in hyperglycemic patients. Fundamental and Clinical Pharmacology. 2009;**23**:501-507. DOI: 10.1111/j.1472-8206.2009.00700.x

[111] Sahana DA, Shivaprakash G, Baliga R, Prabha A, Ganesh J, Pai MR. Effect of *Eugenia jambolana* on plasma glucose, insulin sensitivity and HDL-C levels: Preliminary results of a randomized clinical trial. Journal of Pharmacy Research. 2010;**3**:1268-1270

[112] Ayya N, Nalwade V, Khan TN. Effect of Jamun (*Syzygium cumini* L.) seed powder supplementation on blood glucose level of type-II diabetic subject. Food Science Research Journal. 2015;**6**:353-356. DOI: 10.15740/HAS/FSRJ/6.2/353-356

[113] Banu H, Jyothi A. Hypoglycemic and hypocholesterolemic effect of *Eugenia jambolana* (kala jamun) spicy mix on type II diabetic subjects. Imperial Journal of Interdisciplinary Research. 2016;**2**:850-857

[114] Sidana S, Singh VB, Meena BL, Beniwal S, Singh K, Kumar D, et al. Effect of *Syzygium cumini* (jamun) seed powder on glycemic control: A double-blind randomized controlled trial. Journal of the Medical Society. 2017;**31**:185-189. DOI: 10.4103/jms.jms_62_16

[115] Teixeira CC, Rava CA, Mallman da Silva P, Melchior R, Argenta R, Anselmi F, et al. Absence of antihyperglycemic effect of jambolan in experimental and clinical models. Journal of Ethnopharmacology. 2000;**71**:343-347. DOI: 10.1016/s0378-8741(00)00185-9

[116] Teixeira CC, Fuchs FD, Weinert LS, Esteves J. The efficacy of folk medicines in the management of type 2 diabetes mellitus: Results of a randomized controlled trial of *Syzygium cumini* (L.) Skeels. Journal of Clinical Pharmacy and Therapeutics. 2006;**31**:1-5. DOI: 10.1111/j.1365-2710.2006.00700.x

[117] Chatham-Stephens K, Taylor E, Chang A, Peterson A, Daniel J, Martin C, et al. Hepatotoxicity associated with weight loss or sports dietary supplements, including OxyELITE Pro™—United States, 2013. Drug Testing and Analysis. 2017;**9**:68-74. DOI: 10.1002/dta.2036

[118] Roy SK, Sing RN. Bael fruit (*Aegle marmelos*): A potential fruit for processing. Economic Botany. 1979;**33**:203-212

[119] Sharma PC, Bhatia V, Bansal N, Sharma A. A review on bael tree. Natural Product Radiance. 2007;**6**:171-178

[120] Lamia S, Rashed SS, Rashed B, Prima A, Mony A, Dash P. Phytochemistry and pharmacological properties of *Aegle marmelos* L (Rutaceae): A review. International Journal of Pharmacy and Pharmaceutical Sciences. 2018;**3**:45-54

[121] Manandhar B, Paudel KR, Sharma B, Karki R. Phytochemical profile and pharmacological activity of *Aegle marmelos* Linn. Journal of Integrative Medicine. 2018;**16**:153-163. DOI: 10.1016/j.joim.2018.04.007

[122] Thokchom DS, Singh AR. Ethnopharmacological relevance of *Aegle marmelos* (L.) Correa for treatment of diabetes mellitus: A review. International Journal of Pharmaceutical Sciences Review and Research. 2018;**48**:15-19

[123] Arawwawala LDAM, Jayaratne DLSM. *Aegle marmelos* (L.) Correa as a potential candidate for treatment of diabetes mellitus: A review Journal of Herbmed Pharmacology 2017;6:141-147

[124] Sharma B, Satapathi SK, Roy P. Hypoglycemic and hypolipidemic effect of *Aegle marmelos* (L.) leaf extract on streptozotocin-induced diabetic mice. International Journal of Pharmacology. 2007;**3**:444-452. DOI: 10.3923/ijp.2007.444.452

[125] Arumugama S, Kavimanib S, Kadalmanic B, Ahmedd ABA, Akbarshac MA, Rao MA. Antidiabetic activity of leaf and callus extracts of *Aegle marmelos* in rabbit. ScienceAsia. 2008;**34**:317-321. DOI: 10.2306/scienceasia1513-1874.2008.34.317

[126] Bhavani R. Antidiabetic activity medicinal plant *Aegle marmelos* (Linn.) on alloxan induced diabetic rats. International Research Journal of Pharmaceutical and Biosciences. 2014;**1**:36-44

[127] Mudi SR, Akhter M, Biswas SK, Muttalib MA, Choudhury S, Rokeya B, et al. Effect of aqueous extract of *Aegle marmelos* fruit and leaf on glycemic, insulinemic and lipidemic status of type 2 diabetic model rats. Journal of Complementary and Integrative Medicine. 2017;**14**:20160111. DOI: 10.1515/jcim-2016-0111

[128] Sabu MC, Kuttan R. Antidiabetic activity of *Aegle marmelos* and its relationship with its antioxidant properties. Indian Journal of Physiology and Pharmacology. 2004;**48**:81-88

[129] Abdallah IZA, Salem IS, Abd El-Salam NAS. Evaluation of antidiabetic and antioxidant activity of *Aegle marmelos* L. Correa fruit extract in diabetic rats. Egyptian. Journal of Hospital Medicine. 2017;**67**:731-741

[130] Upadhya S, Shanbhag KK, Suneetha G, Balachandra Naidu M, Upadhya S. A study of hypoglycemic and antioxidant activity of *Aegle marmelos* in alloxan induced diabetic rats. Indian Journal of Physiology and Pharmacology. 2004;**48**:476-480

[131] Siddique NA, Mujeeb M, Ansari SH, Ahmad S, Ali B, Aslam J. Development of quality standards of *Aegle marmelos* leaves. Journal of Phytology. 2010;**2**:36-43

[132] Ahmad W, Amir M, Ahmad A, Ali A, Ali A, Wahab S, et al. P. *Aegle marmelos* leaf extract phytochemical analysis, cytotoxicity, *in vitro* antioxidant and antidiabetic activities. Plants. 2021;**10**:2573. DOI: 10.3390/plants10122573

[133] Ogata M, Hoshi M, Urano S, Endo T. Antioxidant activity of eugenol and related monomeric and dimeric compounds. Chemical and Pharmaceutical Bulletin. 2000;**48**:1467-1469. DOI: 10.1248/cpb.48.1467

[134] Sharma BR, Rattan RK, Sharma P. Marmeline an alkaloid and other components of unripe fruits of *Aegle marmelos*. Phytochemistry. 1981;**20**:2606-2607

[135] Vimal V, Devaki T. Linear furanocoumarin protects rat myocardium against lipid peroxidation and membrane damage during experimental myocardial injury. Biomedicine and Pharmacotherapy. 2004;**58**:393-400. DOI: 10.1016/j.biopha.2003.12.007

[136] Kumar V, Ahmed D, Verma A, Anwar F, Ali M, Mujeeb M. Umbelliferone β-D-galactopyranoside from *Aegle marmelos* (L.) Corr. An ethnomedicinal plant with antidiabetic, antihyperlipidemic and antioxidative activity. BMC Complementary and Alternative Medicine. 2013;**13**:273. DOI: 10.1186/1472-6882-13-273

[137] Panaskar SN, Joglekar MM, Taklikar SS, Haldavnekar VS,

Arvindekar AU. *Aegle marmelos* Correa leaf extract prevents secondary complications in streptozotocin-induced diabetic rats and demonstration of limonene as a potent antiglycating agent. Journal of Pharmacy and Pharmacology. 2013;**65**:884-894. DOI: 10.1111/jphp.12044

[138] Phuwapraisirisan P, Puksasook T, Jong-Aramruang J, Kokpol U. Phenylethyl cinnamides: A new series of alpha-glucosidase inhibitors from the leaves of *Aegle marmelos*. Bioorganic and Medicinal Chemistry Letters. 2008;**18**:4956-4958. DOI: 10.1016/j.bmcl.2008.08.024

[139] Sankhla A, Sharma S, Sharma N. Hypoglycemic effect of bael patra (*Aegle marmelos*) in NIDDM patients. Asian Journal of Dairy and Food Research. 2009;**28**:233-236

[140] Singh U, Kochhar A. Effect of supplementation of bael (*Aegle marmelos* L.) and nutrition counseling on blood glucose, lipid profile and blood pressure of non-insulin-dependent diabetics. Journal of Pharma Research. 2012;**1**:1-6. DOI: 10.5281/zenodo.1098649

[141] Sharma K, Shukla S, Chauhan ES. Evaluation of *Aegle marmelos* (Bael) as hyperglycemic and hyperlipidemic diminuting agent in type II diabetes mellitus subjects. The Pharma Innovation Journal. 2016;**5**:43-46

[142] Ismail MYM. Clinical evaluation of antidiabetic activity of Trigonella seeds and *Aegle marmelos* leaves. World Applied Sciences Journal. 2009;**7**:1231-1234

[143] Aziz M, Akhter M. Effect of *Aegle marmelos* fruit pulp powder on glycemic status of type 2 diabetic patients. Ibrahim Medical College Journal. 2013;**7**:35-37. DOI: 10.3329/imcj.v7i2.20109

[144] Ong HC, Norzalina J. Malay herbal medicine in Gemencheh, Negeri Sembilan, Malaysia. Fitoterapia. 1999;**70**:10-14

[145] Samuel AJ, Kalusalingam A, Chellappan DK, Gopinath R, Radhamani S, Husain HA, et al. Ethnomedical survey of plants used by the Orang Asli in Kampung Bawong, Perak, West Malaysia. Journal of Ethnobiology and Ethnomedicine. 2010;**6**:5. DOI: 10.1186/1746-4269-6-5

[146] Koay YC, Wong KC, Osman H, Eldeen IMS, Asmawi MZ. Chemical constituents and biological activities of *Strobilanthes crispus* L. Records of Natural Products. 2013;**7**:59-64

[147] Norfarizan-Hanoon NA, Asmah R, Rokiah MY, Fauziah O, Faridah H. Effects of *Strobilanthes crispus* juice on wound healing and antioxidant enzymes in normal and streptocotocin-induced diabetic rats. Journal of Biological Sciences. 2009;**9**:1727-3048. DOI: 10.3923/jbs.2009.662.668

[148] Nurraihana H, Norfarizan-Hanoon NA. Phytochemistry, pharmacology and toxicology properties of *Strobilanthes crispus*. International Food Research Journal. 2013;**20**(5):2045-2056

[149] Ghasemzadeh A, Jaafar HZ, Rahmat A. Phytochemical constituents and biological activities of different extracts of *Strobilanthes crispus* (L.) Bremek leaves grown in different locations of Malaysia. BMC Complementary and Alternative Medicine. 2015;**15**:422. DOI: 10.1186/s12906-015-0873-3

[150] Hartanti D, Budipramana K. Traditional antidiabetic plants from Indonesia. Ethnobotany Research and Applications. 2020;**19**:34. DOI: 10.32859/era.19.34.1-24

[151] Fadzelly AB, Asmah R, Fauziah O. Effects of *Strobilanthes crispus* tea aqueous extracts on glucose and lipid profile in normal and streptozotocin-induced hyperglycemic rats. Plant Foods for Human Nutrition. 2006;**61**:7-12. DOI: 10.1007/s11130-006-0002-z

[152] Lim KT, Lim V, Chin JH. Subacute oral toxicity study of ethanolic leaves extracts of *Strobilanthes crispus* in rats. Asian Pacific Journal of Tropical Biomedicine. 2012;**2**:948-952. DOI: 10.1016/S2221-1691(13)60005-2

[153] Norfarizan-Hanoon NA, Asmah R, Fauziah O, Rokiah MY, Faridah H. Absence of toxicity of *Strobilanthes crispus* juice in acute oral toxicity study in Sprague dawley rats. Journal Sains Malaysiana. 2012;**41**:403-409

[154] Norfarizan-Hanoon N, Asmah R, Rokiah M, Fauziah O, Faridah H. Antihyperglycemic, hypolipidemic and antioxidant enzymes effect of *Strobilanthes crispus* juice in normal and streptozotocin-induced diabetic male and female rats. International Journal of Pharmacology. 2009;**5**:200-207. DOI: 10.3923/ijp.2009.200.207

[155] Al-Henhena N, Mahmood AA, Al-magrami A, Nor Syuhada AB, Zahra AA, Summaya MD, et al. Histological study of wound healing potential by ethanol leaf extract of *Strobilanthes crispus* in rats. Journal of Medicinal Plants Research. 2011;**5**:3660-3666

[156] Ismail M, Manickam E, Danial AM, Rahmat A, Yahaya A. Chemical composition and antioxidant activity of *Strobilanthes crispus* leaf extract. Journal of Nutritional Biochemistry. 2000;**11**:536-542. DOI: 10.1016/s0955-2863(00)00108-x

[157] Liza MS, Rahman RA, Mandana B, Jinap S, Rahmat A, Zaidul ISM, et al. Supercritical carbon dioxide extraction of bioactive flavonoid from *Strobilanthes crispus* (pecah kaca). International Food Research Journal. 2012;**19**:503-508

[158] Obolskiy D, Pischel I, Siriwatanametanon N, Heinrich M. *Garcinia mangostana* L.: A phytochemical and pharmacological review. Phytotherapy Research. 2009;**23**:1047-1065. DOI: 10.1002/ptr.2730

[159] Xie Z, Sintara M, Chang T, Ou B. Daily consumption of a mangosteen-based drink improves *in vivo* antioxidant and anti-inflammatory biomarkers in healthy adults: A randomized, double-blind, placebo-controlled clinical trial. Food Science and Nutrition. 2015;**3**:342-348. DOI: 10.1002/fsn3.225

[160] Lobb AL. Science in liquid dietary supplement promotion: The misleading case of mangosteen juice. Hawaii Journal of Medicine and Public Health. 2012;**71**:46-48

[161] Chairat M, Bremner J, Kan C. Dyeing of cotton and silk yarn with the extracted dye from the fruit hulls of mangosteen, *Garcinia mangostana* Linn. Fibers and Polymers. 2007;**8**:613-619. DOI: 10.1007/BF02875998

[162] Pedraza-Chaverri J, Cárdenas-Rodríguez N, Orozco-Ibarra M, Pérez-Rojas JM. Medicinal properties of mangosteen (*Garcinia mangostana*). Food and Chemical Toxicology. 2008;**46**:3227-3239. DOI: 10.1016/j.fct.2008.07.024

[163] Ovalle-Magallanes B, Eugenio-Pérez D, Pedraza-Chaverri J. Medicinal properties of mangosteen (*Garcinia mangostana* L.): A comprehensive update. Food and Chemical Toxicology. 2017;**109**:102-122. DOI: 10.1016/j.fct.2017.08.021

[164] Rizaldy D, Hartati R, Nadhifa T, Fidrianny I. Chemical compounds and pharmacological activities of mangosteen (*Garcinia mangostana* L.)—Updated review. Biointerface Research in Applied Chemistry. 2022;**12**:2503-2516. DOI: 10.33263/BRIAC122.25032516]

[165] Yoshimura M, Ninomiya K, Tagashira Y, Maejima K, Yoshida T, Amakura Y. Polyphenolic constituents of the pericarp of mangosteen (*Garcinia mangostana* L.). Journal of Agricultural and Food Chemistry. 2015;**63**:7670-7674. DOI: 10.1021/acs.jafc.5b01771

[166] Chin YW, Kinghorn AD. Structural characterization, biological effects, and synthetic studies on xanthones from mangosteen (*Garcinia mangostana*), a popular botanical dietary supplement. Mini-Reviews in Organic Chemistry. 2008;**5**:355-364. DOI: 10.2174/157019308786242223

[167] Yang R, Li P, Li N, Zhang Q, Bai X, Wang L, et al. Xanthones from the pericarp of *Garcinia mangostana*. Molecules. 2017;**22**:1-10. DOI: 10.3390/molecules22050683

[168] Taher M, Tg Zakaria TM, Susanti D, Zakaria ZA. Hypoglycaemic activity of ethanolic extract of *Garcinia mangostana* Linn. in normoglycaemic and streptozotocin-induced diabetic rats. BMC Complementary and Alternative Medicine. 2016;**16**:135. DOI: 10.1186/s12906-016-1118-9

[169] Karim N, Rahman A, Chanudom L, Thongsom M, Tangpong J. Mangosteen vinegar rind from *Garcinia mangostana* prevents high-fat diet and streptozotocin-induced type II diabetes nephropathy and apoptosis. Journal of Food Science. 2019;**84**:1208-1215. DOI: 10.1111/1750-3841.14511

[170] Karim N, Rahman MA, Changlek S, Tangpong J. Short-time administration of xanthone from *Garcinia mangostana* fruit pericarp attenuates the hepatotoxicity and renotoxicity of type II diabetes mice. Journal of the American College of Nutrition. 2020;**39**:501-510. DOI: 10.1080/07315724.2019.1696251

[171] Adiputro D, Widodo M, Romdoni R, Sargowo D. Extract of mangosteen increases high density lipoprotein levels in rats fed high lipid. Universa Medicina. 2015;**32**:37-43

[172] Abuzaid AS, Sukandar EY, Kurniati NF, Adnyana IK. Antihyperlidemic effects of mangosteen (*Garcinia mangostana* L.) pericarp ethanolic extract in high-carbohydrate Wistar rats. Journal of Natural Remedies. 2017;**17**:165-173. DOI: 10.18311/jnr/2017/11051

[173] Mekseepralard C, Areebambud C, Suksamrarn S, Jariyapongskul A. Effects of long-term α-mangostin supplementation on hyperglycemia and insulin resistance in type 2 diabetic rats induced by high fat diet and low dose streptozotocin. Journal of the Medical Association of Thailand. 2015;**98**:S23-S30

[174] Lee D, Kim YM, Jung K, Chin YW, Kang KS. Alpha-mangostin improves insulin secretion and protects INS-1 cells from streptozotocin-induced damage. International Journal of Molecular Sciences. 2018;**19**:1484. DOI: 10.3390/ijms19051484

[175] Bumrungpert A, Kalpravidh RW, Chuang CC, Overman A, Martinez K, Kennedy A, et al. Xanthones from mangosteen inhibit inflammation in human macrophages and in human adipocytes exposed to macrophage-conditioned media. Journal of Nutrition. 2010;**140**:842-847. DOI: 10.3945/jn.109.120022

[176] Loo AE, Huang D. Assay-guided fractionation study of alpha-amylase

inhibitors from *Garcinia mangostana* pericarp. Journal of Agricultural and Food Chemistry. 2007;**55**:9805-9810. DOI: 10.1021/jf071500f

[177] Ryu HW, Cho JK, Curtis-Long MJ, Yuk HJ, Kim YS, Jung S, et al. Alpha-glucosidase inhibition and antihyperglycemic activity of prenylated xanthones from *Garcinia mangostana*. Phytochemistry. 2011;**72**:2148-2154. DOI: 10.1016/j.phytochem.2011.08.007

[178] Ibrahim SRM, Mohamed GA, Khayat MTA, Ahmed S, Abo-Haded H. α-Amylase inhibition of xanthones from *Garcinia mangostana* pericarps and their possible use for the treatment of diabetes with molecular docking studies. Journal of Food Biochemistry. 2019;**43**:1-9. DOI: 10.1111/jfbc.12844

[179] Udani JK, Singh BB, Barrett ML, Singh VJ. Evaluation of mangosteen juice blend on biomarkers of inflammation in obese subjects: A pilot, dose finding study. Nutrition Journal. 2009;**8**:48. DOI: 10.1186/1475-2891-8-48

[180] Stern JS, Peerson J, Mishra AT, Sadasiva Rao MV, Rajeswari KP. Efficacy and tolerability of a novel herbal formulation for weight management. Obesity. 2013;**21**:921-927. DOI: 10.1002/oby.20211

[181] Watanabe M, Gangitano E, Francomano D, Addessi E, Toscano R, Costantini D, et al. Mangosteen extract shows a potent insulin sensitizing effect in obese female patients: A prospective randomized controlled pilot study. Nutrients. 2018;**10**:586. DOI: 10.3390/nu10050586

[182] Becker LC, Bergfeld WF, Belsito DV, Hill RA, Klaassen CD, Liebler DC, et al. Safety assessment of Panax spp root-derived ingredients as used in cosmetics. International Journal of Toxicology. 2015;**34**:5S-42S. DOI: 10.1177/1091581815610508

[183] Yang CG. The history and origin of notoginseng. Research and Practice in Chinese Medicine. 2015;**29**:83-86

[184] Wang T, Guo R, Zhou G, Zhou X, Kou Z, Sui F, et al. Traditional uses, botany, phytochemistry, pharmacology and toxicology of *Panax notoginseng* (Burk.) F.H. Chen: A review. Journal of Ethnopharmacology. 2016;**188**:234-258. DOI: 10.1016/j.jep.2016.05.005

[185] Ratan ZA, Haidere MF, Hong YH, Park SH, Lee J-O, Lee J, et al. Pharmacological potential of ginseng and its major component ginsenosides. Journal of Ginseng Research. 2021;**45**:199-210. DOI: 10.1016/j.jgr.2020.02.004

[186] Mehta SD, Rathore P, Rai G. Ginseng: Pharmacological action and phytochemistry prospective. In: Hano C, Chen J, editors. Ginseng—Modern Aspects of the Famed Traditional Medicine [Working Title]. London: IntechOpen; 2021. DOI: 10.5772/intechopen.99646

[187] Leung KW, Wong AS. Pharmacology of ginsenosides: A literature review. Chinese Medicine. 2010;**5**:20. DOI: 10.1186/1749-8546-5-20

[188] Yang X, Xiong X, Wang H, Wang J. Protective effects of *Panax notoginseng* saponins on cardiovascular diseases: A comprehensive overview of experimental studies. Evidence-based Complementary and Alternative Medicine. 2014;**2014**:204840. DOI: 10.1155/2014/204840

[189] Bai L, Gao J, Wei F, Zhao J, Wang D, Wei J. Therapeutic potential of ginsenosides as an adjuvant treatment for diabetes. Frontiers in

Pharmacology. 2018;**9**:423. DOI: 10.3389/fphar.2018.00423

[190] Zhou B, Zhang G, Guo W, Ren C, Li M. Xiaoke decoction in treatment of type II diabetes: A meta-analysis. Chinese Herbal Medicines. 2022;**14**:130-141. DOI: 10.1016/j.chmed.2021.08.004

[191] Gong YH, Jiang JX, Li Z, Zhu LH, Zhang ZZ. Hypoglycemic effect of sanchinoside C1 in alloxan-diabetic mice. Yao Xue Bao (Acta Pharmaceutica Sinica). 1991;**26**:81-85

[192] Chen ZH, Li J, Liu J, Zhao Y, Zhang P, Zhang MX, et al. Saponins isolated from the root of *Panax notoginseng* showed significant anti-diabetic effects in KK-Ay mice. American Journal of Chinese Medicine. 2008;**36**:939-951. DOI: 10.1142/S0192415X08006363

[193] Yang CY, Wang J, Zhao Y, Shen L, Jiang X, Xie ZG, et al. Anti-diabetic effects of *Panax notoginseng* saponins and its major anti-hyperglycemic components. Journal of Ethnopharmacology. 2010;**130**:231-236. DOI: 10.1016/j.jep.2010.04.039

[194] Guo X, Sun W, Luo G, Wu L, Xu G, Hou D, et al. *Panax notoginseng* saponins alleviate skeletal muscle insulin resistance by regulating the IRS1-PI3K-AKT signaling pathway and GLUT4 expression. FEBS Open Bio. 2019;**9**:1008-1019. DOI: 10.1002/2211-5463.12635

[195] Zhang X, Zhang B, Zhang C, Sun Guibo Sun X. Effect of *Panax notoginseng* saponins and major anti-obesity components on weight loss. Frontiers in Pharmacology. 2021;**11**:601751. DOI: 10.3389/fphar.2020.601751

[196] Kim JJ, Xiao H, Tan Y, Wang ZZ, Paul Seale J, Qu X. The effects and mechanism of saponins of *Panax notoginseng* on glucose metabolism in 3T3-L1 cells. American Journal of Chinese Medicine. 2009;**37**:1179-1189. DOI: 10.1142/S0192415X09007582

[197] Huang X, Liu G, Guo J, Su Z. The PI3K/AKT pathway in obesity and type 2 diabetes. International Journal of Biological Sciences. 2018;**14**:1483-1496. DOI: 10.7150/ijbs.27173

[198] Fan Y, Qiao Y, Huang J, Tang M. Protective effects of *Panax notoginseng* saponins against high glucose-induced oxidative injury in rat retinal capillary endothelial cells. Evidence-Based Complementary and Alternative Medicine. 2016;**2016**:5326382. DOI: 10.1155/2016/5326382

[199] Liang MT, Lau WY, Sokmen B, Spalding TW, Chuang WJ. Effects of *Panax notoginseng* (Chinese ginseng) and acute exercise on postprandial glycemia in non-diabetic adults. Journal of Complementary and Integrative Medicine. 2012;**8**:/j/jcim.2011.8.issue-1/1553-3840.1402/1553-3840.1402.xml. DOI: 10.2202/1553-3840.1402

[200] Tang X, Huang M, Jiang J, Liang X, Li X, Meng R, et al. *Panax notoginseng* preparations as adjuvant therapy for diabetic kidney disease: A systematic review and meta-analysis. Pharmaceutical Biology. 2020;**58**:138-145. DOI: 10.1080/13880209.2020.1711782

[201] Shi Y, Wan X, Shao N, Ye R, Zhang N, Zhang Y. Protective and anti-angiopathy effects of ginsenoside Re against diabetes mellitus via the activation of p38 MAPK, ERK1/2 and JNK signaling. Molecular Medicine Reports. 2016;**14**:4849-4856. DOI: 10.3892/mmr.2016.5821

[202] Heghes SC, Vostinaru O, Mogosan C, Miere D, Iuga CA, Filip L. Safety profile of nutraceuticals rich

in coumarins: An update. Frontiers in Pharmacology. 2022;**13**:803338. DOI: 10.3389/fphar.2022.803338

[203] Hamidpour R, Hamidpour M, Hamidpour S, Shahlari M. Cinnamon from the selection of traditional applications to its novel effects on the inhibition of angiogenesis in cancer cells and prevention of Alzheimer's disease, and a series of functions such as antioxidant, anticholesterol, antidiabetes, antibacterial, antifungal, nematicidal, acaracidal, and repellent activities. Journal of Traditional and Complementary Medicine. 2015;**5**:66-70. DOI: 10.1016/j.jtcme.2014.11.008

[204] Zhang C, Fan L, Fan S, Wang J, Luo T, Tang Y, et al. *Cinnamomum cassia* Presl: A review of its traditional uses, phytochemistry, pharmacology and toxicology. Molecules. 2019;**24**:3473. DOI: 10.3390/molecules24193473

[205] Wang J, Su B, Jiang H, Cui N, Yu Z, Yang Y, et al. Traditional uses, phytochemistry and pharmacological activities of the genus *Cinnamomum* (Lauraceae): A review. Fitoterapia. 2020;**146**:104675. DOI: 10.1016/j.fitote.2020.104675

[206] Kwon KB, Kim EK, Jeong ES, Lee YH, Lee YR, Park JW, et al. Cortex cinnamomi extract prevents streptozotocin- and cytokine-induced beta-cell damage by inhibiting NF-kappaB. World Journal of Gastroenterology. 2006;**12**:4331-4337. DOI: 10.3748/wjg.v12.i27.4331

[207] Lu Z, Jia Q, Wang R, Wu X, Wu Y, Huang C, et al. Hypoglycemic activities of A- and B-type procyanidin oligomer-rich extracts from different cinnamon barks. Phytomedicine. 2011;**18**:298-302. DOI: 10.1016/j.phymed.2010.08.008

[208] Kim SH, Hyun SH, Choung SY. Anti-diabetic effect of cinnamon extract on blood glucose in db/db mice. Journal of Ethnopharmacology. 2006;**104**:119-123. DOI: 10.1016/j.jep.2005.08.059

[209] Li J, Liu T, Wang L, Guo X, Xu T, Wu L, et al. Antihyperglycemic and antihyperlipidemic action of cinnamaldehyde in C57BLKS/J db/db mice. Journal of Traditional Chinese Medicine. 2012;**32**:446-452. DOI: 10.1016/s0254-6272(13)60053-9

[210] Verspohl EJ, Bauer K, Neddermann E. Antidiabetic effect of *Cinnamomum cassia* and Cinnamomum zeylanicum *in vivo* and *in vitro*. Phytotherapy Research. 2005;**19**:203-206. DOI: 10.1002/ptr.1643

[211] Uslu GA, Gelen V, Uslu H, Özen H. Effects of *Cinnamomum cassia* extract on oxidative stress, immunereactivity of iNOS and impaired thoracic aortic reactivity induced by type II diabetes in rats. Brazilian Journal of Pharmaceutical Sciences. 2018;**54**:e17785. DOI: 10.1590/s2175-97902018000317785

[212] Rao PV, Gan SH. Cinnamon: A multifaceted medicinal plant. Evidence-Based Complementary and Alternative Medicine. 2014;**2014**:642942. DOI: 10.1155/2014/642942

[213] Roussel AM, Hininger I, Benaraba R, Ziegenfuss TN, Anderson RA. Antioxidant effects of a cinnamon extract in people with impaired fasting glucose that are overweight or obese. Journal of the American College of Nutrition. 2009;**28**:16-21. DOI: 10.1080/07315724.2009.10719756

[214] Adisakwattana S, Lerdsuwankij O, Poputtachai U, Minipun A, Suparpprom C. Inhibitory activity of cinnamon bark species and their combination effect with acarbose against intestinal α-glucosidase and

pancreatic α-amylase. Plant Foods for Human Nutrition. 2011;**66**:143-148. DOI: 10.1007/s11130-011-0226-4

[215] Kang BH, Racicot K, Pilkenton SJ, Apostolidis E. Evaluation of the *in vitro* anti-hyperglycemic effect of *Cinnamomum cassia* derived phenolic phytochemicals, via carbohydrate hydrolyzing enzyme inhibition. Plant Foods for Human Nutrition. 2014;**69**:155-160. DOI: 10.1007/s11130-014-0415-z

[216] Ercan P, El SN. Inhibitory effects of bioaccessible anthocyanins and procyanidins from apple, red grape, cinnamon on α-amylase, α-glucosidase and lipase. International Journal for Vitamin and Nutrition Research. 2021;**91**:16-24. DOI: 10.1024/0300-9831/a000652

[217] Couturier K, Qin B, Batandier C, Awada M, Hininger-Favier I, Canini F, et al. Cinnamon increases liver glycogen in an animal model of insulin resistance. Metabolism. 2011;**60**:1590-1597. DOI: 10.1016/j.metabol.2011.03.016

[218] Mang B, Wolters M, Schmitt B, Kelb K, Lichtinghagen R, Stichtenoth DO, et al. Effects of a cinnamon extract on plasma glucose, HbA, and serum lipids in diabetes mellitus type 2. European Journal of Clinical Investigation. 2006;**36**:340-344. DOI: 10.1111/j.1365-2362.2006.01629.x

[219] Allen RW, Schwartzman E, Baker WL, Coleman CI, Phung OJ. Cinnamon use in type 2 diabetes: An updated systematic review and meta-analysis. Annals of Family Medicine. 2013;**11**:452-459. DOI: 10.1370/afm.1517

[220] Hlebowicz J, Darwiche G, Björgell O, Almér LO. Effect of cinnamon on postprandial blood glucose, gastric emptying, and satiety in healthy subjects. American Journal of Clinical Nutrition. 2007;**85**:1552-1556. DOI: 10.1093/ajcn/85.6.1552

[221] Solomon TP, Blannin AK. Effects of short-term cinnamon ingestion on *in vivo* glucose tolerance. Diabetes, Obesity and Metabolism. 2007;**9**:895-901. DOI: 10.1111/j.1463-1326.2006.00694.x

[222] Solomon TP, Blannin AK. Changes in glucose tolerance and insulin sensitivity following 2 weeks of daily cinnamon ingestion in healthy humans. European Journal of Applied Physiology. 2009;**105**:969-976. DOI: 10.1007/s00421-009-0986-9

[223] Wang J, Wang S, Yang J, Henning SM, Ezzat-Zadeh Z, Woo S-L, et al. Acute effects of cinnamon spice on post-prandial glucose and insulin in normal weight and overweight/obese subjects: A pilot study. Frontiers in Nutrition. 2021;7:619782. DOI: 10.3389/fnut.2020.619782

[224] Magistrelli A, Chezem JC. Effect of ground cinnamon on postprandial blood glucose concentration in normal-weight and obese adults. Journal of the Academy of Nutrition and Dietetics. 2012;**112**:1806-1809. DOI: 10.1016/j.jand.2012.07.037

[225] Vanschoonbeek K, Thomassen BJ, Senden JM, Wodzig WK, van Loon LJ. Cinnamon supplementation does not improve glycemic control in postmenopausal type 2 diabetes patients. Journal of Nutrition. 2006;**136**:977-980. DOI: 10.1093/jn/136.4.977

[226] Wickenberg J, Lindstedt S, Nilsson J, Hlebowicz J. *Cassia cinnamon* does not change the insulin sensitivity or the liver enzymes in subjects with impaired glucose tolerance. Nutrition Journal. 2014;**13**:96. DOI: 10.1186/1475-2891-13-96

[227] Gutierrez JL, Bowden RG, Willoughby DS. *Cassia cinnamon* supplementation reduces peak blood glucose responses but does not improve insulin resistance and sensitivity in young, sedentary, obese women. Journal of Dietary Supplements. 2016;**13**:4614-4671. DOI: 10.3109/19390211.2015.1110222

Chapter 2

Hypoglycemia and Brain: The Effect of Energy Loss on Neurons

Daniel Arturo Martínez-Piña,
Gustavo Alexis Alvarado-Fernández,
Edith González-Guevara, Carlos Castillo-Pérez,
Gerardo Romero-Luna and Jorge Alejandro Torres-Ríos

Abstract

Glucose provides the necessary fuel to cover the physiological functions of the organism. In the brain, glucose represents the main energy supply through the generation of adenosine triphosphate, with oxygen and glucose being the main components involved. The imbalance in glucose levels in the central nervous system produces substantial changes in metabolism. Hypoglycemia, or decreased blood glucose levels below 50 mg/dl, is accompanied by symptoms such as decreased performance of cognitive tasks such as verbal fluency, reaction time, arithmetic ability, verbal memory and visual, in addition to excitotoxicity, oxidative stress, neuroinflammation and apoptosis. Hyperglycemia participates in some cardiovascular diseases, neuropathy, nephropathy, retinopathy. Changes in glucose metabolism must be regulated and considered in order to obtain the best treatment for different pathologies, such as infections, non-infections, traumatic, primary or acquired.

Keywords: hyperglycemia, hypoglycemia, neuroglycopenia, neuroinflammation, oxidative stress

1. Introduction

The human brain requires a high and continuous input of energy, which is obtained mainly from glucose, due to its high metabolic rate. Some interesting facts about the brain are that it accounts for only 2% of body weight, but it also requires 15% of cardiac output, 20% of total body oxygen and 25% of serum glucose, which means that the human brain uses up between 5 and 10 g of glucose per hour or 140 g per day on average [1]. Under normal conditions, serum glucose is around 80–90 mg/dl and may increase up to 200 mg/dl after meals. On the other hand, serum glucose may decrease up to 54 mg/dl during prolonged fasting. The concept of hypoglycemia refers to a clinical situation in which patients have a serum glucose value below 50 mg/dl matching with neuroglycopenic symptoms or serum glucose values below 40 mg/dl without any symptoms [1]. The high energy requirements of the human brain employ such complex metabolic strategies to manage energy sources. Glucose enters the central nervous system through the Blood-Brain Barrier (BBB), a process that requires a transport protein located in the cell membrane [2, 3]. There are two systems of glucose and other monosaccharide transporter proteins: sodium-glucose transporters, also known as SGLTs (sodium-dependent glucose transport), and glucose transporters, also known as GLUTs (glucose transporters). There are several types of GLUT transporters in the human body, but in the central nervous system, there are only two types: GLUT1, which is found in the BBB, and GLUT3, which is found in neurons. Glucose enters cells via GLUT transporters in a process composed of four steps; (1) first, glucose binds to the transporter protein on the outer face of the cell membrane; (2) the transporter protein changes its conformation and glucose enters into the cell membrane; (3) glucose is released into the cytoplasm by the transporter; (4) the transporter returns to its original conformation and its glucose binding site is exteriorized again (**Figure 1**) [4, 5].

The human brain requires a lot of energy to carry out all its functions, this energy comes from different pathways in which glucose and oxygen work together to develop adenosine triphosphate (ATP). The bonds of the ATP molecule are then broken to obtain stored energy, and most of this energy is used for information processing. For example, in the human brain, there are about 10 billion neuronal cells communicated by more than 50 trillion synapses through neurotransmitters that are synthesized in the cerebral cortex in a process that requires about 3.8 × 1012 molecules of ATP [5, 6].

Neuronal and glial cells have distinct functions and are metabolically different from each other [6]. In fact, the gray matter of the human brain uses 10 times more glucose than any other organ in the body. With the known stoichiometry of glucose oxidation ($C_6H_{12}O_6$ + $6O_2$ $6CO_2$ + $6H_2O$) and its coupled reactions, it is possible to obtain an estimated flux at different points in the metabolic chain. This allows us to know how glucose enters into glycolysis and the Krebs cycle, leading to the release of energy that is then split into small components such as ATP, increasing its molar flux to 31 molecules of ATP for each molecule of glucose [7].

Oxidation of glucose molecules through the tricarboxylic acid cycle develops small amounts of lactate, which plays an important role as a precursor to the process of

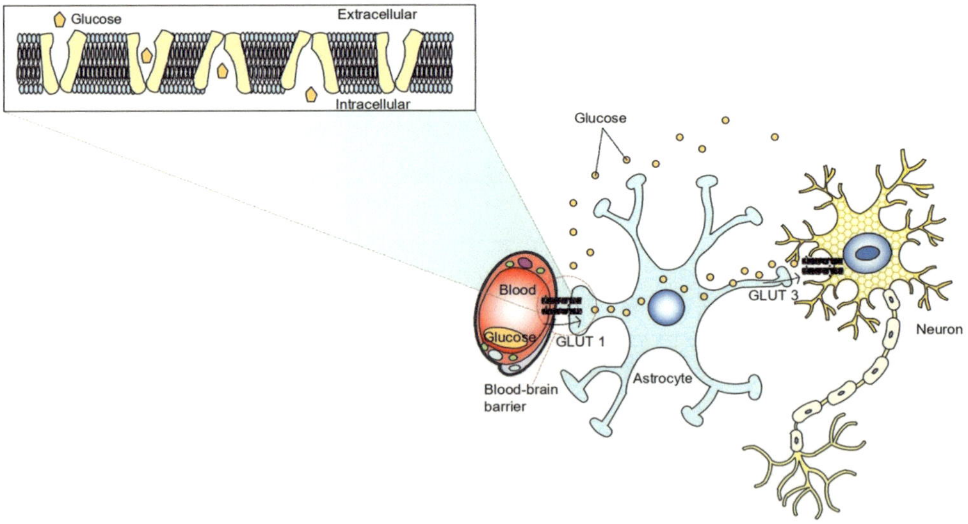

Figure 1.
Glucose transport from blood vessels to neuronal cells. GLUT (glucose transporters). Modified from Iatreia: 2002;15(3).

gluconeogenesis in the nervous system. Lactate becomes an energetic compound for the nervous system, which is demonstrated in neuronal and glial uptake, improving ATP synthesis in neurons. Such articles suggest that glucose is stored by the astrocytes and then released as glucose or lactate, to be used by neurons, when energetic requirements increase [8].

2. Cellular and molecular facts of glucose

Glucose is absorbed by GLUT1 protein transporters and can be stored as glycogen (the most important storage of glycogen is located on astrocytes) or go into glycolysis (**Figure 2**) [9].

2.1 Neurons

Glucose represents the main source of energy and its metabolic regulation is so important for normal nerve cell functions, including ATP synthesis, regulation of oxidative stress, synthesis of neurotransmitters and neuromodulatory molecules and many processes such as memory, learning and sensitivity and motor functions [10, 11]. The overall performance of neurons, astrocytes and endothelial cells is very important during the transit of energy supplements in the nervous system necessary to cover cellular functions [12]. As mentioned above, neuronal cells require a high amount of energy which is obtained from glucose; also glucose can be obtained directly by neurons or indirectly from astrocytes that converted lactate into glucose previously [13, 14]. In normal conditions, neurons obtain energy from glucose, but

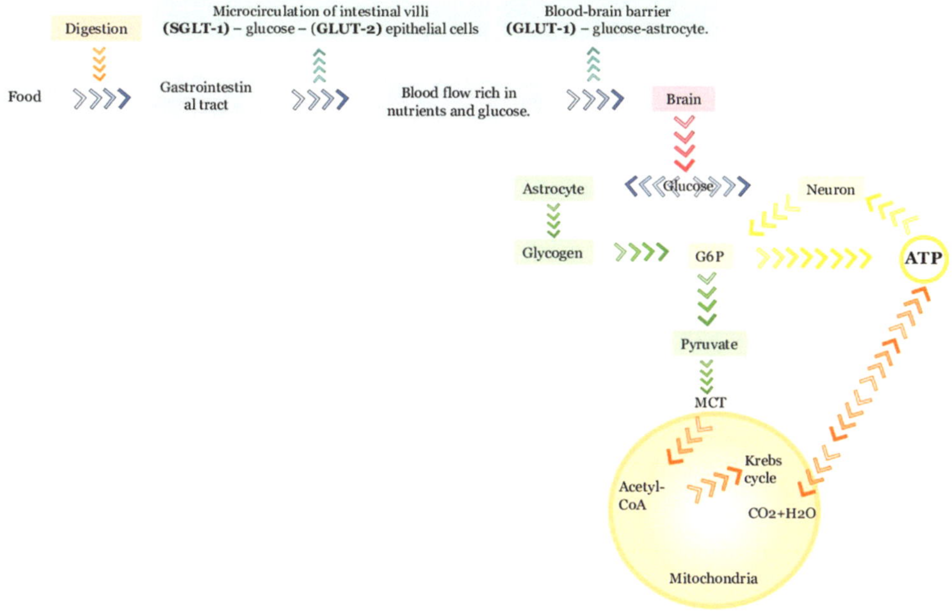

Figure 2.
Pathway of glucose from food to ATP in the neuron. The blue color is the area outside the blood-brain barrier, the green color represents only processes in the astrocyte, the yellow color processes in the neuron, and the orange color represents the intramitochondrial pathways.

during the synaptic activity, they mainly consume lactate as a product of glucose metabolism. In both cases, the overall net brain consumption would be sustained by glucose. Under conditions of glutamatergic synaptic activity, glutamate stimulates GLUT-1-mediated glucose incorporation and glycolysis in astrocytes, followed by the release of lactate into the extracellular space and its capture in neurons, the neuron uptake of glucose is made via the GLUT-3 transporter [9, 15–17].

2.2 Astrocytes

Astrocytes also need the energy to carry out their functions, these cells play such an important role in brain metabolism by providing lactate as a metabolic substrate when neuronal energy requirements increase. In astrocyte cells, the GLUT-1 transport protein is the main glucose uptake protein. Once glucose enters the astrocyte, it is converted to glucose-6-phosphate (G6P) to undergo glycolysis or be converted to glycogen. Glucogenic enzymes involved in glycogen metabolism, such as glycogen synthase, store backup glycogen. Glycogen phosphorylase and the debranching enzyme metabolize glycogen into G6P to undergo glycolysis when the astrocyte, or near neurons, require energy sources (**Figure 3**) [18, 19].

2.3 Hypoglycemia in neurons and astrocytes

It has been described that hypoglycemia actively causes neuronal death. When glucose concentration decreases below 1 mM (18 mg/dl), causes energy deficit, the release of excitatory amino acids (aspartate and glutamate) induces the expression of

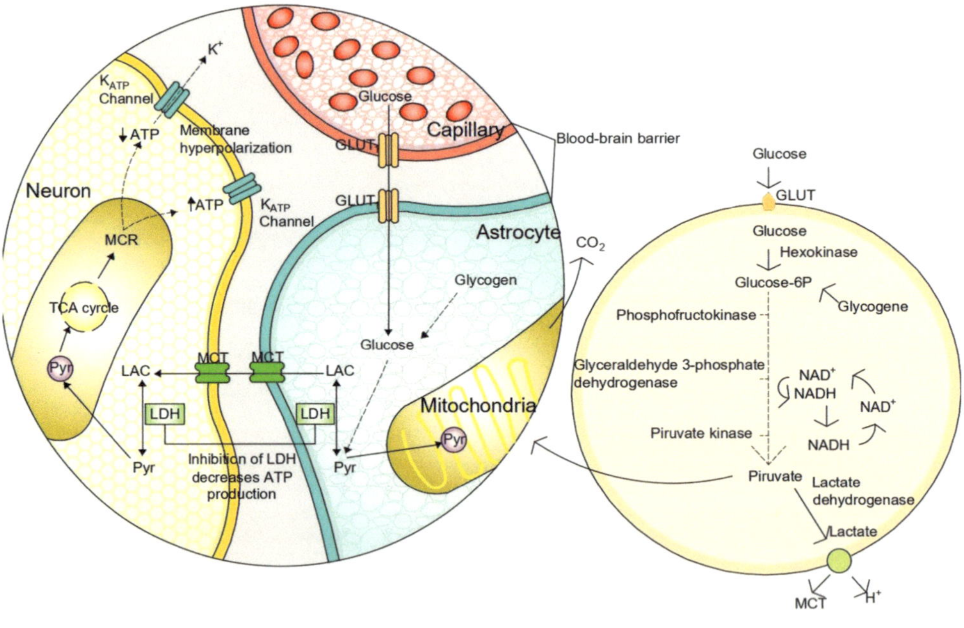

Figure 3.
Glucose metabolism and energy synthesis in astrocytes and neurons. LDH (lactate dehydrogenase), MCT (medium-chain triglycerides), LAC (lactate), ATP (adenosine triphosphate), NAD+ (nicotinamide adenine dinucleotide oxidized), NADH (nicotinamide adenine dinucleotide reduced), H+ (hydrogen), Pyr (pyruvate). Modified from N Engl J Med 2015; 373:187–189.

excitatory receptors located in neuronal dendrites that produce calcium fluxes, inducing neuronal necrosis. Hypoglycemia constitutes a metabolic brain injury [20, 21].

During hypoglycemia or periods of intense brain activity, glycogen can be used to generate lactate, which is translocated to nearby neuronal cells. Thus, glycogen within astrocytes functions as a backup system in case of hypoglycemia, ensuring neuronal functions and survival during glucose deprivation [22, 23]. In cases of brain ischemia, astrocytes have shown a high resistance, a situation that is explained by its glycogen store. Astrocytes also keep glucose synthesis for longer time periods compared with neuronal cells. Besides, astrocytes lead glycogen to turn into lactate which is moved within neurons when these cells have increased energy requirements or during lack of glucose. However, the amount of mitochondria within astrocyte cells is smaller than the amount of mitochondria within neuronal cells. A single molecule of lactate can generate 10 mM ATP, which is equivalent to 17 molecules of ATP [7, 23]. Several papers suggest that glucose molecules are stored mainly in astrocyte cells and can be released as glucose or lactate to contribute to neuronal metabolism when energy needs increase [8, 22, 23]. Other studies, recently published, suggest that other substrates such as pyruvate, glycogen, ketone bodies, glutamate, glutamine and aspartate can be metabolized by neuronal cells in case of glucose deprivation, supporting neuronal functions and delaying ATP depletion during hypoglycemia [24]. Astrocytes can release purines made of adenine, specifically adenosine (which plays an important role as a neuroprotective molecule) and guanosine which can lead to cell repair after a brain injury (**Figure 3**) [25].

In situations of low glycogen levels, glycogen can modulate some neurotransmitters and also serum glucose levels. These facts are explained by the fact that, during periods of hypoglycemia, glycogen is converted into lactate and reaches nearby neurons and axons where it is used as an energy source, leading to protection against hypoglycemia-induced brain injury and ensuring that neuronal functions supplying energy demands [26].

3. Cellular and molecular neuroglycopenia

3.1 Calcium and hypoglycemic damage

As mentioned above, intracellular calcium accumulation promotes lipolysis, increasing the amount of free fatty acids due to phospholipids metabolism, including arachidonic acid, activated by cyclooxygenase enzyme and promoting oxygen reactive species releasing, platelet aggregation and neutrophil chemotaxis, leading to inflammation and direct/indirect cell damage. Calcium accumulation can also activate regulatory mechanisms to keep adequate levels of this ion, such as calsequestrin and chelation promoted by the endoplasmic reticulum and mitochondria [27]. When these mechanisms fail, an ionic overcharge takes place in the mitochondria and the cell membrane polarity is dropped. When the membrane potential is dispelled, the ATP synthase works upside down, metabolizing ATP. Also, it is impossible to generate ATP by Krebs cycle or oxidative phosphorylation. Serum calcium levels decrease during isoelectric periods and return to normal levels after glucose administration. This fact correlates to an increase in intracellular calcium levels and neuronal injury. Besides, proapoptotic factors are released as cytochrome C, caspase 3 and apoptosis-inducing factors. A persistent state of oxidative stress

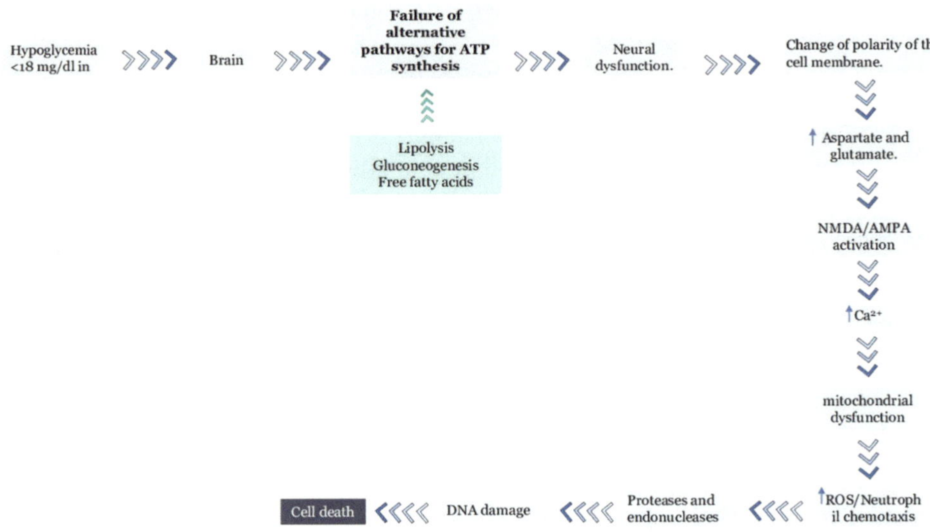

Figure 4.
Example of severe hypoglycemia in the brain.

is induced by a failure in the I and IV complex of the electron transport chain and release of reactive oxygen species (**Figure 4**) [28].

3.2 Reactive oxygen species and oxidative stress

Oxygen ions, free radicals and peroxides are very small molecules, which appear as a result of oxygen metabolism, and play an important role in the oxidation-reduction process, activating genes, exchanging ions when their values need to be regulated. The regulating mechanisms to avoid over synthesis of these small molecules include important enzymes groups such as catalase and superoxide dismutase. There are also antioxidant molecules, for example, ascorbic acid, uric acid and glutathione. Oxidative stress can be defined as a metabolic status with overproduction of oxygen reactive species and exceeding the antioxidant molecules' capacity to offset this process. Some important molecules that can be affected by this situation are cell membrane lipids, deoxyribonucleic acid (DNA) and proteins. An increase in catalase and superoxides dismutase enzymes indicate, indirectly, the presence of peroxides and superoxide, respectively. That is because these enzymes are considered important indirect markers of oxidative stress [29].

The glutathione tripeptide functions as a chemical synthesis buffer during oxidation-reduction reactions carried out by the mitochondria. This chemical buffer is made of glycine, glutamate and cysteine. Another chemical buffer that appears in cases of oxidative stress is glutathione in its oxidized form, which is formed by two glutathione molecules linked by a disulfide bond. There is also an increase in nitric oxide synthase, subsequently, nitric oxide becomes reactive when it is combined with superoxides, forming peroxynitrite, a highly reactive molecule with a short half-life, which in addition to oxidizing nearby molecules, can be transformed into nitrotyrosine when reacting with tyrosine residues, increasing immunoreactivity. The neuronal cells located on the Ammon's horn 1 region (CA1), in the hippocampus, promote an increase in zinc levels during long times of hypoglycemia. The glucose reintroduction

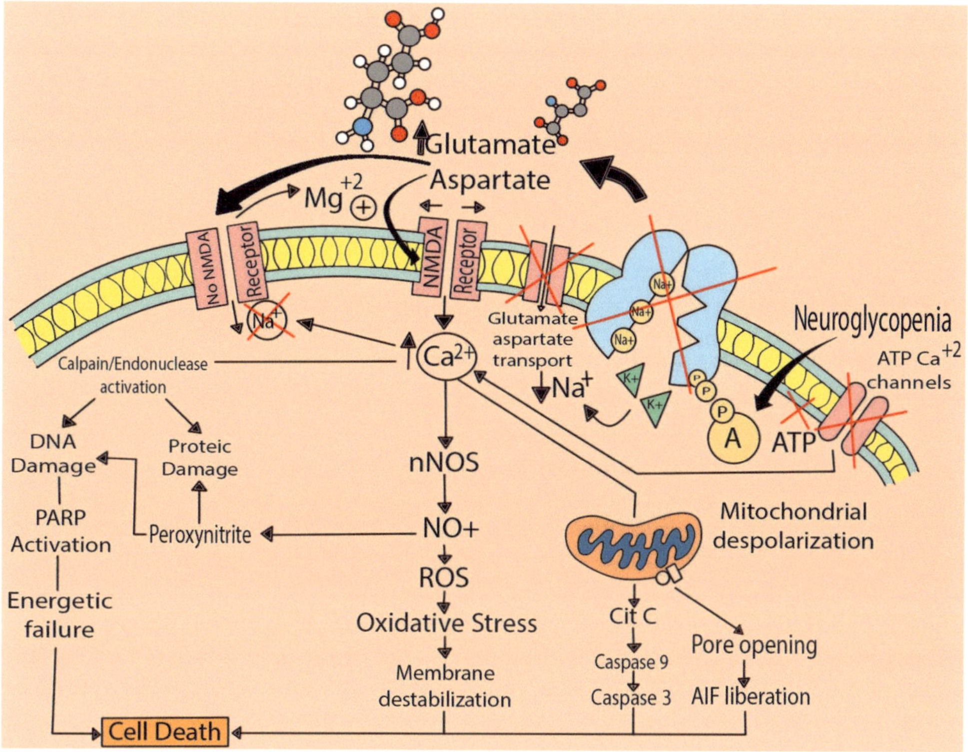

Figure 5.
Cell death in neuroglycopenia. DNA (deoxyribonucleic acid), PARP (poly-ADPribose), NMDA (N-methyl-D-aspartate), Mg² (magnesium), Ca2⁺ (calcium), Na⁺ (sodium), K⁺ (potassium), nNOS (neuronal nitric oxide synthase), NO+ (derived from oxygen species), ROS (reactive oxygen species), Cit C (cytochrome C), AIF (apoptosis inducing factor).

to the system promotes zinc vesicles and nitric oxide synthesis that trigger neuronal damage. Zinc activates the NADPH enzyme oxidase (NOX) and poly-ADP ribose (PARP-1) after being translocated to postsynaptic neurons, leading to the production of reactive oxygen species (ROS), depletion of oxidized nicotinamide adenine dinucleotide (NAD+) and lead to neuronal death. The production of ROS by NOS and NOX induces DNA damage and consequent activation of PARP-1, which consumes the NAD+ which is required for glucose oxidation through the glycolytic pathway, as well as activating programmed cell death pathways such as calpain [30]. During hypoglycemia, PARP-1 activation is an important factor involved in neuronal death (it leads to increased nitrotyrosine and products of this polymerase). On the other hand, PARP-1 inhibitors can rescue neurons that would otherwise die after severe hypoglycemia (**Figures 4** and **5**) [31, 32].

3.3 Apoptosis and inflammatory response

Apoptosis is a type of cell death that depends on energy and various cellular functions in which the membrane retains its integrity. For its activation, specific proteins are required to avoid inflammatory responses, which are divided into intrinsic and extrinsic pathways. The intrinsic activation pathway consists of caspases and calpain. Caspases are classified as initiators, such as caspase 9 and executors, including caspase 3. The intrinsic pathway starts with the release of cytochrome C from the mitochondrial inner membrane, which increases its concentration in the cytosol and binds APAF1 (apoptotic protease-activating factor 1) protein, dATP and procaspase 9 zymogen [29, 32]. Once bound, this complex becomes an active initiator form of the pathway, caspase 9, which consequently causes the activation of the executioner pathway, procaspases 3 and 7, responsible for promoting apoptosis.

It has been postulated recently that an inflammatory response also participates in hypoglycemic cell damage, this is known due to a study that demonstrates microglial reactivity in the rat of hippocampus 1–7 days after 30 minutes of hypoglycemic isoelectric, with activation of calpain, xanthine oxidase and phospholipase A2.

Tkacs and cols., demonstrated that three hypoglycemic episodes related to 30–35 mg/dl glucose blood levels increased the number of positive cells to TUNEL (apoptosis marker in the arcuate nucleus of the hypothalamus). Subsequently, other authors reported positive degenerative cells to the neuronal death marker Fluoro-Jade B (FJB) after only 1 week of a single hypoglycemia event, particularly in the cerebral cortex, although some were also observed in the hippocampus and striatum [33].

In 1880, blood glucose levels were measured for the first time, which made it possible to understand the different clinical neurological manifestations and their association with low blood glucose levels [34]. It was in 1938, when the surgeon Allen Whipple proposed a triad characterized by hypoglycemia symptoms, decreased venous glucose concentration and the disappearance of these symptoms after the correction of glycemia. Although this description was proposed as criteria to perform or not the insulinomas resection, this triad became widely generalized among the medical community in the face of hypoglycemia events due to any cause. Reversibility of the clinical syndrome is frequent when treatment is initiated, although there are also less fortunate scenarios in which sustained damage to the nervous system is produced, which will depend on the degree of hypoglycemia when treatment is not timely. This situation is directly related to functional prognosis and mortality [34, 35].

The physician must be able to identify the clinical signs of hypoglycemia since the first organ to suffer the consequences is the brain, and we must avoid unfavorable outcomes, such as neuronal damage and death (neuroglycopenia). When the arterial glucose supply is interrupted and the protective mechanisms are overcome, the previously described alterations occur at the level of ionic gradients, neurotransmitter release and reuptake, and oxidative stress, culminating in mitochondrial and cellular dysfunction [36].

There are usually very effective endogenous mechanisms to prevent neuroglycopenia. The first line of defense against falling blood glucose levels is to decrease endogenous insulin production, increasing hepatic glucose production and decreasing its utilization by other peripheral tissues such as muscle and fat tissue [37]. If glucose levels remain low, there will be glucagon secretion, followed by an increase in adrenaline. These counterregulatory mechanisms will be as intense as hypoglycemia severity, resulting in mobilization of glycogen stores, gluconeogenesis and decreased glucose utilization at the peripheral level [38].

A very particular characteristic of the brain is the high consumption of glucose and oxygen, with a high tolerance to periods of transient deficit of these substrates, however, when glucose decreases below 20 mg/dl, there is a cessation of brain electrical activity (hypoglycemic coma). Blood glucose concentrations may decrease to 30% of the normal value, but this supply must be constant, as neuronal glycogen stores are limited and depleted in less than 2 minutes. From this point on, the extent of neuronal damage is directly related to the time the isoelectric period is maintained. Neuronal death occurs after a period of approximately 15 minutes of inactivity. Repeated episodes of hypoglycemia cause irreversible damage, causing the irreversible cognitive deficit, which correlates to various brain structures, the most sensitive to the damage being the cortex, hippocampus and striatum [39].

3.4 Excitatory amino acids in hypoglycemic damage

Excitotoxicity refers to the ability of some amino acids (glutamate) to cause neurodegeneration secondary to prolonged stimulation of postsynaptic receptors. This type of toxicity was first described in cerebral vascular disease; later evidence was found in severe hypoglycemia. The mechanism of damage is as follows: extracellular concentrations of glutamate are regulated by reuptake into the synaptic space by specific transporters located in astrocytes and neurons. This reuptake is mediated by sodium, regulated by the electrochemical gradient of ATP-dependent Na/K+ pumps. These ionotropic receptors are classified according to their specific agonist: the N-methyl D-aspartate (NMDA) receptor, permeable to calcium and sodium. The non-NMDA receptors (kainate receptor and a-amino-3-hydroxy-methyloxazole-4propionic acid (AMPA) are sensitive to sodium [40].

Under resting conditions, the NMDA receptor ion channel is blocked by magnesium, which is released during depolarization mediated by non-NMDA aspartate receptor-dependent ion channels, allowing calcium to enter the intracellular space. Both glutamate and aspartate have been shown to be associated with neuronal damage in hypoglycemia, being released in large amounts during the isoelectric trace [41]. In this situation glutamate is used as a metabolic substrate, favoring the release of aspartate by altering the electrochemical gradient of Na+/K+, promoting the accumulation of intracellular calcium and with it, the release of vesicles by exocytosis with excitatory neurotransmitters. Even with the accumulation of excitatory neurotransmitters, the inhibition of their transporters can limit neurological damage; however, when there is an absence of energetic substrates, neuronal death is induced. As mentioned, neuronal death and cognitive impairment caused by hypoglycemia suggest that they are involved in excitotoxicity and DNA damage.

4. Neuroglycopenia secondary to hypoglycemia

To avoid neuronal death during a period of hypoglycemia, the brain sets in motion two main regulatory mechanisms: increased cerebral blood flow and the use of alternative substrate pools to glucose [39, 41]. During hypoglycemia, oxygen consumption remains constant, giving rise to the theory that these alternative pools are able to compensate for the lack of glucose, allowing adequate cellular function during relatively short periods of hypoglycemia. The brain can use other substrates for energy, such as lactate, pyruvate and ketone bodies, although the primary substrate in the first instance appears to be glycogen, which seems to be depleted in more than 5 minutes after the onset of the isoelectric period [42].

The nervous system is very susceptible to changes when serum glycemia value is low, which leads to protective mechanisms; on the other hand, when there is hyperglycemia it has a better regulation. The endocrine counterregulatory response mechanisms that are activated when glucose drops below 70 mg/dl, at the level of the pancreatic b-cells the first response is initiated, which consists in the cessation of insulin release and when the glucose level reaches 66 mg/dl, growth hormone and cortisol are released, which stimulate lipolysis in adipose tissue, ketogenesis and gluconeogenesis in the liver. Below 54 mg/dl, glucagon (a hormone produced in pancreatic cells, which stimulates hepatic glucose production through glycogenolysis and gluconeogenesis) and epinephrine are secreted. Epinephrine secreted by the adrenal glands increases glycogenolysis and gluconeogenesis in the liver, stimulates lipolysis and decreases insulin secretion while elevating glucagon release (**Table 1**) [38, 39, 42].

The first modulatory process in hypoglycemia is decreased insulin synthesis. This is followed by an increase in other involved hormones such as GH, ACTH, glucagon, and epinephrine, resulting in the activation of metabolic regulatory pathways such as lipolysis, ketogenesis, and gluconeogenesis.

Recurrent hypoglycemia can cause the loss of these counterregulatory mechanisms and create a vicious cycle increases the risk of severe hypoglycemia with each event. Recurrent hypoglycemia reduces the glucose levels necessary to trigger the autonomic counterregulatory response during a subsequent hypoglycemic period, leading to patients being unable to recognize sympathoadrenal symptoms, leading to the onset of neuroglycopenic symptoms (hypoglycemia unawareness). The unawareness of hypoglycemia and the failure of the autonomic response lead to the so-called hypoglycemia-associated autonomic failure, which increases the risk of severe hypoglycemia by 25 times or more, with high chances of coma, irreversible brain damage and death. Clinical data suggest that about 25% of diabetic patients suffer hypoglycemia without realizing it [37, 39, 42]. Hypoglycemia occurs in 25–30% of diabetic patients, with type 1 diabetics being more affected, followed by type 2 diabetics, although in them it usually happens in advanced stages of the disease. The incidence of hypoglycemia episodes depends on the age and duration of the disease. The mortality rate is between 4 and 10% and is attributable to severe hypoglycemia in type 1 diabetic patients with the long-standing disease (7–30 years), this is because the continuous administration of insulin or insulin-releasing drugs leads to glucose uptake in fat, muscle and liver, inhibiting gluconeogenesis and glycogenolysis, as well as lipolysis and glucagon secretion from pancreatic cells. As a consequence, the first response to hypoglycemia (inhibition of insulin secretion) is lost, glucagon secretion is suppressed, and epinephrine is secreted at lower glucose levels [37, 38, 42].

4.1 Moderate or severe hypoglycemia

According to histological studies, hypoglycemic coma induces neuronal damage in the cortex, particularly in the insular cortex, hippocampus, caudate nucleus and putamen; lesions have also been identified in the thalamus, globus pallidus and a significant volume decrease in the white matter and gray matter in all cerebral lobes with occipital and parietal predominance. There is a close correlation between the duration of the isoelectric period and the spread of neuronal damage. The most

Organ involved	Response	Effects	
Pancreatic a cells	Decreased insulin synthesis	Blood glucose mobilization is reduced.	
Hypophysis	Increased GH y ACTH	Lipolysis and ketogenesis	Glyconeogenesis
Pancreatic β cells	Increased glucagon	Glycogenolysis	
Adrenal glands	Increased epinephrine and cortisol		

Table 1.
Brain protection mechanisms in neuroglycopenia.

vulnerable brain regions include superficial layers 2 and 3 of the cerebral cortex, CA1, the subiculum and crest of the dentate gyrus, as well as neuronal damage in the dorsolateral region of the striatum [43].

5. Clinical manifestations in neuroglycopenia

Signs and symptoms for hypoglycemia depend on glucose levels (mild, moderate or severe), frequency and duration of episodes. Symptomatology can be divided into two big groups: The first group included sympathoadrenal or neurogenic symptoms due to the activation of the autonomic nervous system and the release of epinephrine and norepinephrine, triggered in moderate hypoglycemia. The symptoms can be hunger, sweating, tingling, tremors, palpitations and anxiety (the initial symptoms that allow the patient to notice the hypoglycemic state). If glucose levels continue dropping to moderate or severe, the patient would develop the second group of symptoms (neuroglycopenic symptoms) which include blurry vision, confusion, dizziness, irritability, bradylalia, lipothymia, drowsiness, bradypsychia, seizures and coma. However, they do not always present the same way, actually, it is one of the first diseases that mimic brain stroke symptoms, among other acute neurologic diseases (hypoglycemic encephalopathy) [34, 35, 44]. Hypoglycemia recurrence induces the body to adapt, and the clinical signs can be minimal or absent until the glucose levels decrease deeply, taking the patient to an impaired consciousness state (**Table 2**) [29, 44].

Mild hypoglycemia has subtle symptoms which are inconspicuous with cognitive changes. Multiple studies have done experiments on both humans and animals, finding an association between hypoglycemia and cognitive impairment, affecting complex abilities more than simple ones, regulated by the hippocampus [45, 46]. After a severe hypoglycemia episode, the cognitive deterioration in different cerebral domains appears in healthy individuals with glucose blood levels between 2.6 and 3.3 mmol/l [47]. Severe hypoglycemia causes a decrease in the performance of cognitive tasks, such as verbal fluency, reaction time, arithmetic abilities and verbal and visual memory [48]. The cognitive function drop is seen after the activation of the counterregulatory response and the presence of neuroglycopenic symptoms in diabetic

Sympathoadrenal symptoms	Neuroglycopenic symptoms	Other symptoms of severe neuroglycopenia
Hunger	Blurred vision	Cognitive changes
Sweating	Confusion	Difficult memory
Paresthesias	Dizziness	Troubles with language
Tremor	Irritability	
Palpitations	Bradylalia	Bradykinesia
Anxiety	Lipothymia	
	Drowsiness	
	Bradypsychia	
	Seizures	
	Coma	

Table 2.
Clinical manifestations of neuroglycopenia.

patients, however, this response changes in non-diabetic patients in whom the cognitive function is immediately impaired, even before the counterregulatory neuroendocrine response starts and senses the neuroglycopenic symptoms (**Table 2**) [47, 48].

In 1990, Ryan et al., evaluated the cognitive effects after a hypoglycemic event in children, using the hypoglycemic clamp technique, with a control group with normal glucose levels. Hypoglycemic values were 3.1–3.6 mmol/l and the euglycemic values were from 5.5 mmol/l onwards, noticing a significant decrease in the trail-making test (mental flexibility), attention and decision making in the mild hypoglycemic group. Also, once the glycemic values were restored (>5.5 mmol/l), there was no recovery observed in the attention or reaction time tests, which suggests a long-term neurological effect [49].

Other studies have documented attention, intelligence and memory disturbances in children with a history of severe hypoglycemia [48, 49]. Childhood hypoglycemia represents an essential factor that affects specific cognitive capabilities such as memory, learning, intelligence and attention, being the most vulnerable cognitive domains to hypoglycemia in children [50, 51]. However, no studies have been made comparing the history of hypoglycemia with long-term control groups, therefore, the sequels that may develop are unknown with certainty.

Also, there have been reported mood disorders associated with repeated events of severe hypoglycemia, especially in depressive disorder until 24 hours after the event. Acute hypoglycemia changes the state of mind causing the patient to feel exhausted and reducing the hedonic tone. The consequence of long-term and repetitive periods of moderate hypoglycemia to neuronal damage and cognitive function is not well understood, however, prolonged hypoglycemia with the absence of isoelectricity can also induce neuron death restricted mainly to the cerebral cortex. Glucose blood concentrations of 30–35 mg/dl for 75 minutes can cause significant neuron damage in the medial prefrontal cortex, piriform cortex and orbital cortex [52].

5.1 Imaging in neuroglycopenia

Objective damage from repeated hypoglycemia events is difficult to document because routine imaging studies are not usually performed in this type of patient, as it is an event that is treated in the emergency room and it usually subsides in a few minutes. However, some studies have evaluated diabetic patients with recurrent hypoglycemia events trying to correlate cognitive alterations and imaging findings in MRI [53]. It has been reported cortical atrophy in type 1 diabetic patients with severe recurrent hypoglycemia events while in patients who do not have recurrent events these findings were not present, nevertheless, these findings were not related to the cognitive alterations. There are also case reports in which the MRI shows a reduction in the white matter of the hippocampus, thalamus and globus pallidus, correlating this with memory loss and anterograde amnesia, however, these findings are not common, which make them statistically insignificant.

6. Neuroglycopenia with and without hypoglycemia in medical scenarios

The physiology of glucose in the human brain has already been discussed thoroughly, its' way through the blood-brain barrier and molecular, cellular, tissue and systemic conditions, on the other hand, it is important to mention some clinical scenarios where these events take place even though there are not evident and can explain part of the symptoms and prognostic in each entity. This section will briefly

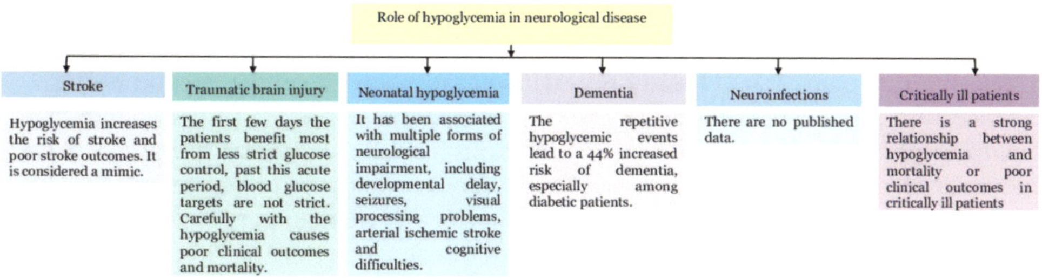

Figure 6.
Hypoglycemia negatively affects diseases of the central nervous system.

describe neuropathologic things that cause glucose levels alterations at the central nervous system and important treatment aspects (**Figure 6**).

6.1 Glucose brain concentration in the intensive care unit

The relationship between changes in glucose values and cardiovascular events, such as stroke and acute myocardial infarction, has been well established. Both hyperglycemia and hypoglycemia are factors that vary patient prognosis [54]. Glucose dysregulation is a common situation in neurocritical patients. Since 1849, the association between hyperglycemia and prognosis has been described in patients with cerebral infarction, a situation that has been repeated in more recent studies [55, 56], which also include patients with acute brain injury secondary to other situations such as meningitis and cranioencephalic trauma [57].

From several years, it has been thought that intensive glucose control by continuous infusion, even to near-normal levels, might be beneficial to the patient; however, the NICE-SUGAR study group conducted a randomized clinical trial comparing intensive glucose control (from 81 to 108 mg/dl) with a group in which glucose levels were more permissive (up to 180 mg/dl), with subcutaneous bolus insulin administration. Glucose below 140 mg/dl was associated with increased hypoglycemia events and increased cardiovascular mortality, whereas glucose levels above 180 mg/dl were associated with the worse neurological recovery and increased likelihood of sequelae [58, 59]. Multiple studies have reached the same conclusion, including the SHINE study, in which intensive control compared with the standard modality did not make a significant difference in functional outcome (Rankin scale at 90 days) [60].

Very loose glucose control was associated with worse neurological recovery, although it does not significantly influence mortality in the neurocritical patient, some sequelae may impact functionality [61].

6.2 Brain glucose concentrations in cerebral infarction

Several clinical trials have shown that cerebral stroke patients with acute elevation of glycemia at the onset of the event suffer worse functional outcomes, longer hospital stay and higher mortality with a higher rate of bleeding after the ischemic event [62]. The definition of hyperglycemia is debated, the reference cohort for different authors usually varies according to the results obtained in clinical trials, where the objective is the correlation between glucose levels and increased mortality, findings are diverse, finding favorable results with levels of 110–155 mg/dl [63, 64]. It has been shown that patients with ischemic stroke who are treated with tissue plasminogen activator benefit from glucose levels below 140 mg/dl in the first hours of treatment, which correlates with the benefit of the fibrinolytic drug, since patients with adequate initial glycemic control had higher reperfusion rates, smaller infarcts, and better functional prognosis than patients with higher glucose levels, this is independent of chronic glycemic dyscontrol [65, 66]. Although evidence indicates that intensive glucose control does not impact mortality, hypoglycemia could have an impact on the development of neurological damage and long-term sequelae, perpetuating the damage already established by previous injuries in the neurocritical patient [67].

6.3 Brain glucose concentrations in patients with traumatic brain injury

During traumatic brain injury there is a net decrease in glucose in microdialysis, but an increase in glutamate and lactate/pyruvate in microdialysis, with an adverse effect on the long-term recovery of neurological function [68]. Care should be taken in the management of these patients, as it is known that during traumatic injury there is hyperglycemia, using insulin to control it and decrease brain damage due to hyperglycemia, however, adequate monitoring should be performed, as lowering glucose levels with insulin may induce and aggravate secondary brain injury [69].

A hypothesis suggests that post-traumatic reductions in extracellular glucose levels are not due to ischemia, but are associated with poor neurological outcomes. Neurosurgical data from the microdialysis catheter in uninjured brain tissue with a perfusion rate of 2 uL/min suggest that glucose values of 0.5–1 mmol/L and lactate of 0.6–1.1 mmol/L are considered normal. In patients with epilepsy versus non-epileptic tissue perfused at 2.5 uL/min, mean glucose values of 0.82 ± 0.27 mmol/L and mean lactate levels of 1.3 ± 0.49 mmol/L were observed [70]. In minimally injured brain trauma patients perfused at a rate of 2 uL/min and under conditions of normal intracranial pressure and normal tissue oxygenation, reports of mean glucose values have ranged from 0.5 to 1.1 mmol/L, demonstrating that glucose variations are not significant during direct trauma [71]. The extracellular glucose level is generally reduced after severe traumatic brain injury and is associated with poor neurological recovery, but is not associated with ischemia [72].

Due to these findings, blood glucose control in patients with traumatic brain injury has recently been the subject of much research [68, 72]. A retrospective study included a total of 228 patients with severe trauma who were treated with insulin. In the first week (acute stage), a blood glucose target of 90–144 mg/dL (5–8 mmol/L) was associated with a reduced mortality rate and a decrease in intracranial pressure (ICP) compared with a blood glucose target of 63–117 mg/dL (3.5–6.5 mmol/L). However, in the second week, the groups appeared to have the reverse results: compared to the target group of 5–8 mmol/L, the 3.5–6.5 mmol/L group demonstrated a lower incidence of ICP and a reduction in infectious complications. Therefore, slightly higher blood glucose (5–8 mmol/L) appears to provide benefits during the first week, whereas lower blood glucose (3.5–6.5 mmol/L) may be more favorable during the later stages of recovery [69, 72]. Another study showed that blood glucose < 6–11 mmol/L could reduce mortality in patients with mild trauma, whereas, in severe cases, the ideal blood glucose target was 7.77–10.0 mmol/L.

Both hyperglycemia and hypoglycemia are harmful [70, 73]. Therefore, methods to improve intensive insulin therapy without inducing secondary complications should be investigated, and attention should also be focused on the prevention of hypoglycemia in patients with head injury [73]. It can be concluded that, in the first few days following traumatic brain injury, patients benefit most from less strict glucose control, and that, past this acute period, blood glucose targets should be modified.

6.4 Hypoglycorrhachia without hypoglycemia

An objective way to demonstrate neuroglycopenia without symptoms is by measuring glucose in the cerebrospinal fluid (CSF). There are multiple etiologies that lower glucose centrally and are recognized not by the symptomatology of neuroglycopenia but by the characteristic symptoms of each disease and the presence of hypoglycorrhachia (there are multiple definitions, however, the most accepted is CSF glucose/serum glucose ratio ≤ 0.5, and < 40 mg/dl is considered severe) [74, 75]. The etiologies are diverse in both children and adults (**Table 3**) [74–76]. Treatment is disease-specific and hypoglycorrhachia is not specifically treated.

6.5 COVID-19

Neuro-COVID has been described for its clinical manifestations and findings in acute neurological disease, and the data that have caused the most impact when talking about encephalitis secondary to COVID-19 is hypoglycorrhachia and changes in the electroencephalogram [77]. Based on the above, our team conducted an investigation during the current SARS-CoV2 pandemic in 30 patients with a diagnosis and positive polymerase chain reaction for SARS-CoV2, without any obvious neurological manifestations, and performed a clinical history, complete physical and neurological examination, lumbar puncture and electroencephalogram, obtaining the following results: We found a high prevalence of minor neurological manifestations, such as headache, anosmia, dysgeusia and hypoaesthesia predominating in the early stages [78]. Other frequent abnormal findings were in the CSF with hypoglycorrhachia >70% and less frequently in the electroencephalogram of the scalp with focal and generalized dysfunction in <20%.

Infectious diseases	Non-infectious diseases
Meningitis caused by typical bacteria, atypical bacteria, viruses, parasites, mycobacteria or fungal etiology.	Carcinomatous meningitis.
	GLUT-1 deficiency syndrome.
Amebic meningoencephalitis.	Leukemia or lymphoma involving CNS.
Cytomegalovirus.	Subarachnoid hemorrhage.
Other causes of hypoglycorrhachia	
Malignant atrophic papulosis.	Neurosarcoidosis.
	Meningitis of rheumatoid etiology.
Cholesterol-induced leptomeningitis.	Behcet's disease.
Rheumatoid meningitis	Dermoid cyst.
Granulomatous angiitis of the central nervous system.	Systemic lupus erythematous with CNS involvement.

Table 3.
Diseases with hypoglycorrhachia without neuroglycopenia.

7. Conclusion

Glucose is the main fuel for the appropriate functioning of the central nervous system. It has been described the main mechanism of entry and use of glucose at the molecular and cellular levels. We emphasize that neurons and astrocytes interact to form common metabolic cooperation generating a neuroprotective effect to avoid hypoglycemic coma or a major brain injury that leads to cellular death. We cannot forget that when a patient has already had neuroglycopenia secondary to hypoglycemia, he/she already has a change in his/her metabolism and recurrence becomes more frequent with each episode, which is why some insulin-dependent diabetics die. The management of glucose in critically ill patients or at the brain level is different and the ideal treatment and glucose values at central and serum levels are not clear. Central nervous system diseases that cause hypoglycorrhachia are treated by etiology and not by low central glucose. Finally, at the time of writing this chapter we faced with the fact that the amount of published information is old and repetitive, it is important to continue research on the damage, prevention and prognosis of glucose levels at the central level in different scenarios.

Acknowledgements

Architect Dulce Maria Gallardo Rocha and Engineer Luis Miguel Vaquera Ortiz for making and editing the images and tables used in this chapter.

Conflict of interest

The authors declare no conflict of interest.

Appendices and nomenclature

AMPA	a-amino-3-hydroxy-methyloxazole-4propionic acid
AIF	apoptosis inducing factor
ATP	adenosine triphosphate
APAF1	apoptotic protease-activating factor 1
BBB	blood brain barrier
Ca2+	calcium
Cit C	cytochrome C
dl	deciliters
DNA	deoxyribonucleic acid
FJB	Fluoro-Jade B
H+	hydrogen
GLUT	glucose transporter
G6P	glucose-6-phosphate
K+	potassium
LAC	(lactate)
LDH	lactate dehydrogenase
MCT	medium-chain triglycerides
mg	milligrams

Mg/dl	milligrams per liter
Mg2	magnesium
mM	millimoles
mmol/l	millimoles per liter
Na+	sodium
NADH	nicotinamide adenine dinucleotide reduced
NAD+	nicotinamide adenine dinucleotide oxidized
NMDA	N-methyl-D-aspartate
nNOS	neuronal nitric oxide synthase
NO+	derived from oxygen species
ROS	reactive oxygen species
SGLT	sodium dependent glucose transport
PARP	poly-ADPribose
Pyr	pyruvate

Author details

Daniel Arturo Martínez-Piña[1*], Gustavo Alexis Alvarado-Fernández[2], Edith González-Guevara[1], Carlos Castillo-Pérez[1], Gerardo Romero-Luna[1] and Jorge Alejandro Torres-Ríos[1]

1 National Institute of Neurology and Neurosurgery, Mexico City, Mexico

2 Hospital Gustavo A Rovirosa Perez, Villahermosa, Mexico

*Address all correspondence to: daniel_264mx@hotmail.com

References

[1] Erbslöh F, Bernsmeier A, Hillesheim H. Der Glucoseverbrauch des Gehirns und seine Abhängigkeit von der Leber. Archiv für Psychiatrie und Nervenkrankheiten. 1958;**196**:611-626

[2] Gruetter EJ, Novotny SD, Boulware DL, Rothman GF, Mason GI, Shulman RG, et al. Direct measurement of brain glucose concentrations in humans by 13C NMR spectroscopy. Proceedings of the National Academy of Science USA. 1992;**89**(3):1109-1112

[3] Gruetter R, Novotny EJ, Boulware SD, Rothman DL, Shulman RG. 1H NMR studies of glucose transport in the human brain. Journal of Cerebral Blood Flow and Metabolism. 1996;**16**(3):427-438

[4] Mayer J. Glucostatic mechanism of regulation of food intake. The New England Journal of Medicine. 1953;**249**:13-16

[5] Carruthers A. Facilitated diffusion of glucose. Physiological Reviews. 1990;**70**:1.135-1.176

[6] Barros LF. Small is fast: Astrocytic glucose and lactate metabolism at cellular resolution. Frontiers in Cellular Neuroscience. 2013;**21**:1-8

[7] Magistretti PJ, Pellerin L. Cellular mechanisms of brain energy metabolism and their relevance to functional brain imaging. Philosophical Transactions of the Royal Society of London. Series B, Biological Sciences. 1999;**354**(1387):1155-1163

[8] Reinstrup P, Ståhl N, Mellergård P, Uski T, Ungerstedt U, Nordström CH. Intracerebral microdialysis in clinical practice: Baseline values for chemical markers during wakefulness, anesthesia, and neurosurgery. Neurosurgery. 2000;**47**(3):701-709

[9] Deitmer JW, Theparambil SM, Ruminot I, Noor SI, Becker H. Energy dynamics in the brain: Contributions of astrocytes to metabolism and pH homeostasis. Frontiers in Neuroscience. 2019;**13**. DOI: 10.3389/fnins.2019.01301

[10] Mergenthaler P, Lindauer U, Dienel GA, Meisel A. Sugar for the brain: The role of glucose in physiological and pathological brain function. Trends in Neurosciences. 2013;**36**(10):587-597

[11] Dienel GA. Brain glucose metabolism: Integration of energetics with function. Physiological Reviews. 2019;**99**(1):949-1045. DOI: 10.1152/physrev.00062.2017

[12] Magistretti PJ, Allaman I. A cellular perspective on brain energy metabolism and functional imaging. Neuron. 2015;**86**(4):883-901

[13] Suzuki A, Stern SA, Bozdagi O, Huntley GW, Walker RH, Magistretti PJ, et al. Astrocyte-neuron lactate transport is required for long-term memory formation. Cell. 2011;**144**(5):810-823

[14] Lundgaard I, Li B, Xie L. Direct neuronal glucose uptake heralds activity-dependent increases in cerebral metabolism. Nature Communications. 2015;**6**:6807-6819

[15] Pellerin L, Magistretti PJ. Glutamate uptake into astrocytes stimulates aerobic glycolysis: A mechanism coupling neuronal activity to glucose utilization Proc. National Academy of Science USA. 1994;**91**:10625-10629

[16] Loaiza A, Porras OH, Barros LF. Glutamate triggers rapid glucose transport

stimulation in astrocytes as evidenced by real-time confocal microscopy. The Journal of Neuroscience. 2003;**23**(19):7337-7342. DOI: 10.1523/JNEUROSCI.23-19-07337.2003

[17] Duelli R, Kuschinsky W. Brain glucose transporters: Relationship to local energy demand. News in Physiological Sciences. 2001;**16**:71-76

[18] Jakoby P, Schmidt E, Ruminot I, Gutiérrez R, Barros LF, Deitmer JW. Higher transport and metabolism of glucose in astrocytes compared with neurons: A multiphoton study of hippocampal and cerebellar tissue slices. Cerebral Cortex. 2014;**24**(1):222-231

[19] Nadeau OW, Fontes JD, Carlson GM. The regulation of glycogenolysis in the brain. The Journal of Biological Chemistry. 2018;**293**(19):7099-7107

[20] Auer RN. Hypoglycemic brain damage. Metabolic Brain Disease. 2004;**19**:169-175

[21] De Angelis CL, Brigati G, Polleri G, Malova M, Parodi A, Minghetti D, et al. Neonatal hypoglycemia and brain vulnerability. Frontiers in Endocrinology. 2021;**12**:634305-634317

[22] Falkowska A, Gutowska I, Goschorska M, Nowacki P, Chlubek D, Baranowska-Bosiacka I. Energy metabolism of the brain, including the cooperation between astrocytes and neurons, especially in the context of glycogen metabolism. International Journal of Molecular Sciences. 2015;**16**(11):25959-25981

[23] Suh SW, Bergher JP, Anderson CM, Treadway JL, Fosgerau K, Swanson RA. Astrocyte glycogen sustains neuronal activity during hypoglycemia: Studies with the glycogen phosphorylase inhibitor CP-316,819 ([R-R*,S*]-5-chloro-N-[2-hydroxy-3-(methoxymethylamino)-3-oxo-1-(phenylmethyl) propyl]-1H-indole-2-carboxamide). The Journal of Pharmacology and Experimental Therapeutics. 2007 Apr;**321**(1):45-50. DOI: 10.1124/jpet.106.115550

[24] Amaral A. Effects of hypoglycaemia on neuronal metabolism in the adult brain: Role of alternative substrates to glucose. Journal of Inherited Metabolic Disease. 2013;**36**:621-634

[25] Ciccarelli R, Di Iorio P, Giuliani P, D'Alimonte I, Ballerini P, Caciagli F, et al. Rat cultured astrocytes release guanine-based purines in basal conditions and after hypoxia/hypoglycemia. Glia. 1999;**25**(1):93-98

[26] Brown AM, Ransom BR. Astrocyte glycogen and brain energy metabolism. Glia. 2007;**55**(12):1263-1271

[27] Ashfaq M, Moats AR, Northrup H, Singletary CN, Hashmi SS, Koenig MK, et al. Hypoglycemia in mitochondrial disorders. Mitochondrion. 2021;**58**:179-183. DOI: 10.1016/j.mito.2021.03.002

[28] Takata T, Hirai H, Shigemoto T, Okada Y. The release of glutamate and accumulation of intracellular calcium in the guinea pig hippocampal slices during glucose deprivation. Neuroscience Letters. 1995;**189**:21-24

[29] Languren G, Montiel T, Julio-Amilpas A, Massieu L. Neuronal damage and cognitive impairment associated with hypoglycemia: An integrated view. Neurochemistry International. 2013;**63**(4):331-343. DOI: 10.1016/j.neuint.2013.06.018

[30] Páramo B, Hernández-Fonseca K, Estrada-Sánchez A, Jiménez N, Cruz A, Massieu L. Pathways involved

in the generation of reactive oxygen and nitrogen species during glucose deprivation and its role on the death of cultured hippocampal neurons. Neuroscience. 2010;**167**:1057-1069

[31] Suh SW, Aoyama K, Chen Y, Garnier P, Matsumori Y, Gum E, et al. Hypoglycemic neuronal death and cognitive impairment are prevented by poly(ADP-ribose) polymerase inhibitors administered after hypoglycemia. The Journal of Neuroscience. 2003;**23**(33):10681-10690

[32] Won SJ, Jang BG, Yoo BH, Sohn M, Lee MW, Choi BY, et al. Prevention of acute/severe hypoglycemia-induced neuron death by lactate administration. Journal of Cerebral Blood Flow and Metabolism. 2012;**32**(6):1086-1096

[33] Tkacs NC, Dunn-Meynell A, Levin B. Presumed apoptosis and reduced arcuate nucleus nueropeptide Y and pro-opiomelanocortin mRNA in non-coma 1346 hypoglycemia. Diabetes. 2000;**49**:820-826

[34] Mathew P, Thoppil D. Hypoglycemia. StatPearls [Internet] 2021 Available from: https://www.ncbi.nlm.nih.gov/books/NBK534841/ PMID: 30521262. [Accessed: February 15, 2022].

[35] Pourmotabbed G, Kitabchi AE. Hypoglycemia. Obstetrics and Gynecology Clinics of North America. 2001 Jun;**28**(2):383-400

[36] Morgan RK, Cortes Y, Murphy L. Pathophysiology and aetiology of hypoglycaemic crises. The Journal of Small Animal Practice. 2018;**59**(11):659-669. DOI: 10.1111/jsap.12911

[37] Dagogo-Jack S. Hypoglycemia in type 1 diabetes mellitus: Pathophysiology and prevention. Treatments in Endocrinology. 2004;**3**(2):91-103. DOI: 10.2165/00024677-200403020-00004

[38] Yang SW, Park KH, Zhou YJ. The impact of hypoglycemia on the cardiovascular system: Physiology and pathophysiology. Angiology. 2016;**67**(9):802-809. DOI: 10.1177/0003319715623400

[39] Rehni AK, Dave KR. Impact of hypoglycemia on brain metabolism during diabetes. Molecular Neurobiology. 2018;**55**(12):9075-9088. DOI: 10.1007/s12035-018-1044-6

[40] Terpstra M, Moheet A, Kumar A, Eberly LE, Seaquist E, Öz G. Changes in human brain glutamate concentration during hypoglycemia: Insights into cerebral adaptations in hypoglycemia-associated autonomic failure in type 1 diabetes. Journal of Cerebral Blood Flow and Metabolism. 2014;**34**(5):876-882

[41] Honegger P, Braissant O, Henry H, Boulat O, Bachmann C, Zurich MG, et al. Alteration of amino acid metabolism in neuronal aggregate cultures exposed to hypoglycemic conditions. Journal of Neurochemistry. 2002;**51**:1141-1151

[42] Suh SW, Hamby AM, Swanson RA. Hypoglycemia, brain energetics, and hypoglycemic neuronal death. Glia. 2007 Sep;**55**(12):1280-1286

[43] Zoysa N, Rogers H, Choudhary P, Amiel SA, Heller SR, Evans M, et al. Severe hypoglycaemia in type 1 diabetes mellitus: Underlying drivers and potential strategies for successful prevention. Diabetes/Metabolism Research and Reviews. 2014 Mar;**30**(3):175-190. DOI: 10.1002/dmrr.2492

[44] Witsch J, Neugebauer H, Flechsenhar J, et al. Hypoglycemic encephalopathy: A case series and literature review on

outcome determination. Journal of Neurology. 2012;**259**:2172-2181

[45] Xu C, Yogaratman J, Lua R, Naik S, Khoo C, Sasidaran S, et al. Persistent, severe hypoglycemia–induced organic brain syndrome with neurological sequelae: A case report. General Hospital Psichiatry. 2011;**33**:411-412

[46] Cryer PE. Hypoglycemia, functional brain failure, and brain death. Jornal dos Clinicos. 2007;**1035**:868-870

[47] Amiel S. Cognitive function testing in studies of acute hypoglycaemia: Rights and wrongs. Diabetologia. 1998;**41**:713-719

[48] Bakatselos S. Hypoglycemia unawareness. Diabetes Research and Clinical Practice. 2011;**93**:92-96

[49] Ryan C, Atchison J, Puczynski S, Puczynski M, Arslanian S, Becker D. Mild hypoglycaemia associated with deterioration of mental efficiency in children with insulin-dependent diabetes mellitus. The Journal of Pediatrics. 1990;**117**:32-38

[50] Hershey T, Perantie D, Warren SL, Zimmerman EC, Sadler M, White HM. Frequency and timing of severe hypoglycaemia affects spatial memory in children with type 1 diabetes. Diabetes Care. 2005;**28**:2372-2377

[51] Blasetti A, Chiuri R, Tocco A, Di Giulio C, Mattei P, Ballone E, Chiarelli F, Verrotti A. The effect of recurrent severe hypoglycemia on cognitive performance in children with type 1 diabetes: A meta-analysis. Journal of Child Neurology 1000, 2011;**26**:1383-1391

[52] Yaffe K, Falvey CM, Hamilton N. Association between hypoglycemia and dementia in a biracial cohort of older adults with diabetes mellitus. Journal of American Medical Association Internal Medicine. 2013;**173**:1300-1306

[53] Perros P, Deary I, Sellar R, Best JJ, Frier BM. Brain abnormalities demonstrated by magnetic resonance imaging in adult IDDM patients with and without a history of recurrent severe hypoglycemia. Diabetes Care. 1997;**20**:1013-1018

[54] Smith L, Chakraborty D, Bhattacharya P, Sarmah D, Koch S, Dave KR. Exposure to hypoglycemia and risk of stroke. Annals of the New York Academy of Sciences. 2018;**1431**(1):25-34. DOI: 10.1111/nyas.13872

[55] Hernando AM, Gabriel AC. Glycemia in spontaneous intracerebral hemorrhage: Clinical implications, Romanian. Neurosurgery. 2014;**XXI 3**:313-313

[56] Capes SE, Hunt D, Malmberg K, Pathak P, Gerstein HC. Stress hyperglycemia and prognosis of stroke in nondiabetic and diabetic patients: A systematic overview. Stroke. 2001;**32**:2426-2432

[57] Gale SC, Sicoutris C, Reilly PM, Schwab CW, Gracias VH. Poor glycemic control is associated with increased mortality in critically ill trauma patients. The American Surgeon. 2007;**73**:454-460

[58] The NICE-SUGAR Study Investigators. Intensive versus conventional glucose control in critically ill patients. New England Journal of Medicine. 2009;**360**:1283-1297

[59] Oddo M, Schmidt JM, Mayer SA, Chiolero RL. Glucose control after brain injury. Current Opinion in Clinical Nutrition and Metabolic Care. 2008;**11**:134-139

[60] Johnston KC, Bruno A, Pauls Q, Hall CE, Barrett KM, et al. Intensive vs

standard treatment of hyperglycemia and functional outcome in patients with acute ischemic stroke. JAMA. 2019;**322**(4):326. DOI: 10.1001/jama.2019

[61] Kramer AH, Roberts DJ, Zygun DA. Optimal glycemic control in neurocritical care patients: A systematic review and meta-analysis. Critical Care 16, R203 (2012). DOI: 10.1186/cc11812

[62] Hafez S, Coucha M, Bruno A, Fagan SC, Ergul A. Hyperglycemia, acute ischemic stroke, and thrombolytic therapy. Translational Stroke Research. 2014;**5**(4):442-453. DOI: 10.1007/s12975-014-0336-z

[63] Stead LG, Gilmore RM, Bellolio MF, Mishra S, Bhagra A, Vaidyanathan L, et al. Hyperglycemia as an independent predictor of worse outcome in non-diabetic patients presenting with acute ischemic stroke. Neurocritical Care. 2009;**10**:181-186

[64] Fuentes B, Castillo J, San José B, Leira R, Serena J, Vivancos J, et al. Stroke Project of the Cerebrovascular Diseases Study Group, Spanish Society of Neurology. The prognostic value of capillary glucose levels in acute stroke: The Glycemia in Acute Stroke (GLIAS). Study. 2009;**40**:562-568

[65] Masrur S, Cox M, Bhatt DL, Smith EE, Ellrodt G, Fonarow GC, et al. Association of acute and chronic hyperglycemia with acute ischemic stroke outcomes post-thrombolysis: Findings from get with the guidelines-stroke. Journal of the American Heart Association. 2015;**4**:10-23. DOI: 10.1161/jaha.115.002193

[66] Lin S-F, Chao A-C, Hu H-H, Lin R-T, Chen C-H, Chan L, et al. Hyperglycemia predicts unfavorable outcomes in acute ischemic stroke patients treated with intravenous thrombolysis among a Chinese population: A prospective cohort study. Journal of the Neurological Sciences. 2018;**388**:195-202. DOI: 10.1016/j.jns.2018.03.022

[67] Daniel R, Villuri S, Furlong K. Management of hyperglycemia in the neurosurgery patient. Hospital Practice. 2017;**45**(4):150-157. DOI: 10.1080/21548331.2017.1370968

[68] Badjatia N, Vespa P. Monitoring nutrition and glucose in acute brain injury. Neurocritical Care. 2014;**21** (Suppl 2):S159-S167

[69] Meier R, Bechir M, Ludwig S, Sommerfeld J, Keel M, Steiger P, et al. Differential temporal profile of lowered blood glucose levels (3.5 to 6.5 mmol/l versus 5 to 8 mmol/l) in patients with severe traumatic brain injury. Critical Care. 2008;**12**:R98

[70] Abi-Saab WM, Maggs DG, Jones T, Jacob R, Srihari V, Thompson J, et al. Striking differences in glucose and lactate levels between brain extracellular fluid and plasma in conscious human subjects: Effects of hyperglycemia and hypoglycemia. Journal of Cerebral Metabolism. 2002;**22**:271-279

[71] Goodman JC, Valadka AB, Gopinath SP, Uzura M, Robertson CS. Alteraciones extracelulares de lactato y glucosa en el cerebro después de una lesión en la cabeza medida por microdiálisis. Critical Care Medicine. 1999;**27**:1965-1973

[72] Vespa PM, McArthur D, O'Phelan K, Glenn T, Etchepare M, Kelly D, et al. Persistently low extracellular glucose correlates with poor outcome 6 months after human traumatic brain injury despite a lack of increased lactate: A Microdialysis Study. Journal of Cerebral Blood Flow & Metabolism. 2003;**23**(7):865-877. DOI: 10.1097/01.wcb.0000076701.45782

[73] Shi J, Dong B, Mao Y, Guan W, Cao J, Zhu R, et al. Review: Traumatic brain injury and hyperglycemia, a potentially modifiable risk factor. Oncotarget. 2016;**7**(43):71052-71061. DOI: 10.18632/oncotarget.11958

[74] Chow E, Troy SB. The differential diagnosis of hypoglycorrhachia in adult patients. The American Journal of the Medical Sciences. 2014;**348**(3):186-190. DOI: 10.1097/MAJ.0000000000000217

[75] Mohseni S. Neurologic damage in hypoglycemia. Handbook of Clinical Neurology. 2014;**126**:513-532. DOI: 10.1016/b978-0-444-53480-4.00036-9

[76] Arrieta Blanco F, Bélanger Quintana A, Bengoa Rojano N, Stanescu S, MartinezPardo M. Síndrome de deficiencia de GLUT1 y COVID-19 [GLUT1 and COVID-19 deficiency syndrome]. Endocrinology Diabetes Nutrition. 2021;**68**(7):514-515. DOI: 10.1016/j.endinu.2020.07.001

[77] Wu Y, Xu X, Chen Z, et al. Nervous system involvement after infection with COVID-19 and other coronaviruses. Brain, Behavior, and Immunity. 2020;**87**:18-22

[78] Martínez-Piña DA. Neurological characterization in hospitalized patients with COVID 19 in UMAE n° 1 of CMN del Bajio. [thesis]. Universidad Autónoma de Guanajuato; 2021

Section 2

Hypoglycemia: Causes

Chapter 3

Causes of Hypoglycemia

Ala' Abu-Odeh, Dalal Alnatour and Leen Fino

Abstract

Blood glucose levels may vary during the day, when this variation goes below a specific limit, hypoglycemia occurs. Hypoglycemia is often associated with reductions in quality of life and even the risk of death. Moreover, hypoglycemia is correlated with physical and/or psychological morbidity. It is usually a result of the complex interaction between hyperinsulinemia and the compromised physiological and behavioral responses attempting to reduce glucose levels. Nevertheless, several conditions can cause hypoglycemia, both in diabetic and non-diabetic patients. Mutually, diabetic and non-diabetic hypoglycemia is common in terms of several medications, alcohol ingestion, critical illnesses, and non-B cell tumors.

Keywords: hypoglycemia, diabetes, drug-induced hypoglycemia, nondiabetic hypoglycemia

1. Introduction

Glucose is the main source of energy for your body and brain. It can be synthesized de novo or taken from food. Insulin helps to keep blood glucose at normal levels, so your body can work efficiently. Insulin's task is to help glucose to enter your cells and produce energy. If your glucose level is too low, hypoglycemia may occur [1].

Hypoglycemia is defined as a low plasma glucose level of less than 50 mg/dL, thus exposing the subject to potential harm. It is associated with several signs—palpitation, sweating, tremors (adrenergic response), dysarthria, confusion, epilepsy, visual disturbances, and coma (neuroglycopenic response) [2–4]. These affect patients' quality of life and can even increase the risk of death, particularly in diabetic patients. Furthermore, hypoglycemia is often associated with physical and psychological morbidity (such as generalized worry and mood disturbance) [3, 5]. In diabetic patients, the complex interaction between hyperinsulinemia and the compromised physiological and behavioral responses to reduced glucose levels can lead to hypoglycemia [6].

Diabetes—particularly with the use of insulin or sulfonylurea, that is, insulin secretagogue treatment, is the classical cause of hypoglycemia. Moreover, diverse causes are also common, such as medications, alcoholism, critical illness, cachectic state, cortisol insufficiency, gastric or bariatric surgery, pancreas transplantation, glucagon deficiency, dietary toxins, and various conditions (sepsis, starvation, severe excessive exercise), and insulinoma [3, 7, 8]. Not to mention the non-classical causes that may include congenital hyperinsulinism, insulin receptor mutation, inborn errors of metabolism, and non-islet-cell tumor [9].

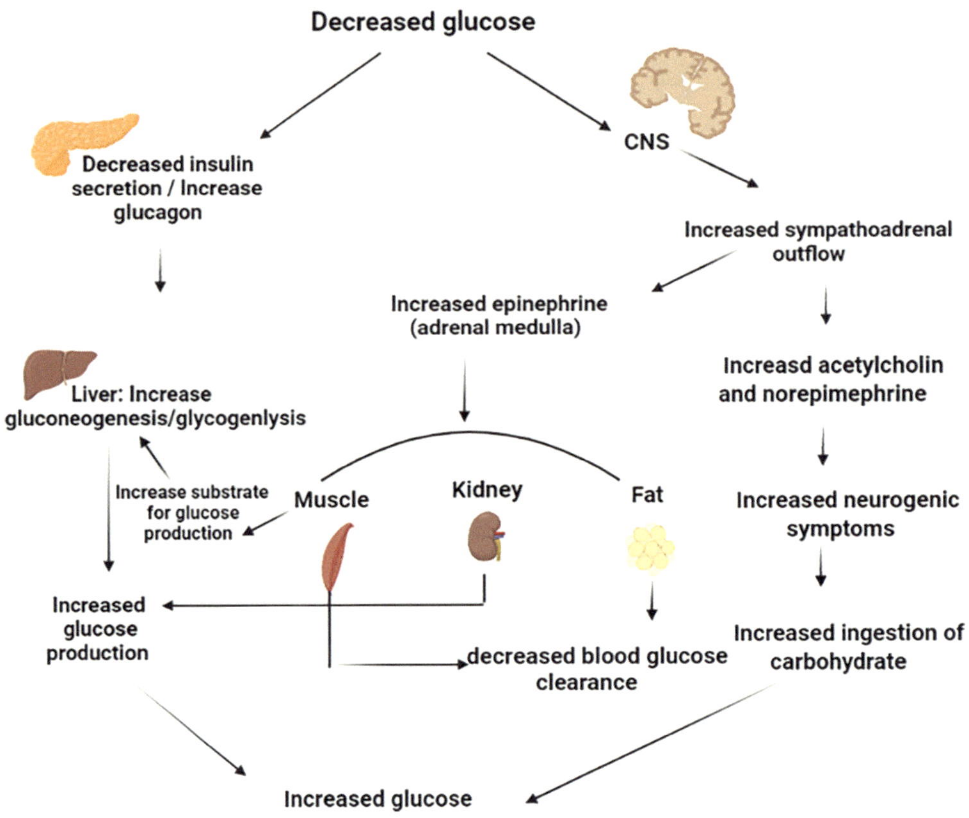

Figure 1.
Physiologic and behavioral defenses against hypoglycemia in humans.

The primary cause of hypoglycemia is a complex interaction between hyperinsulinemia and compromised physiologic and behavioral responses to reducing glucose levels (**Figure 1**).

2. Diabetic hypoglycemia

Diabetic hypoglycemia is both a physiologic and a clinical condition that is associated with increased mortality and morbidity in both type 1 and type 2 diabetes. Hypoglycemia has proven to have detrimental complications for diabetic patients in both the short and long term [10]. There are several causes of hypoglycemia in diabetic patients, including age, renal insufficiency or end-stage renal disease, pregnancy, and polypharmacy of diabetic medications [10, 11], as shown in (**Table 1**).

2.1 Etiology

2.1.1 Drug induced

As mentioned before, hypoglycemia is well known to be associated with diabetes. The risk of hypoglycemia is manifested as a limiting factor and a barrier to optimal treatment and glucose control of type 1 and type 2 diabetes. Although the risk of

Drugs Insulin or insulin secretagogue Alcohol ACEi B-blockers NSAIDs Antimalarials Antibiotics (ciprofloxacin, levofloxacin, gatifloxacin, and moxifloxacin, antiarrhythmics (like quinine, quinidine)) Psychotropic medications	**Insulin related causes** Absolute insulin excess Relative insulin excess a. Exogenous glucose delivery is decreased b. Insulin sensitivity is increased c. Endogenous glucose production is decreased
Malabsorption Celiac disease Pancreatic exocrine insufficiency	**Diabetes complications** Gastroparesis Neuropathy
Hormone deficiency Cortisol Growth hormone Glucagon Epinephrine Hypopituitarism	**Concurrent illness** Renal disease Hepatic disease Cardiac failure Sepsis
Non-islet cell tumor	**Psychological** Fear of hypoglycemia Depression Cognitive impairment

Table 1.
Causes of hypoglycemia in diabetic patients.

hypoglycemia is more common in type 1 diabetes, it is prominent in type 2 diabetes with the use of an insulin secretagogue (such as sulfonylurea and glinides) and insulin [6, 10, 12]. Other types of antidiabetic medications have a low incidence of hypoglycemia.

Drug-induced hypoglycemia is not limited to antidiabetic medication use; other medications can also induce hypoglycemia. The most common non-antihyperglycemic medications that are correlated with hypoglycemia are angiotensin-converting enzyme inhibitors (ACEi), beta-blockers (BB), non-steroidal anti-inflammatory drugs (NSAIDs), antimalarials, antiarrhythmics (such as quinine and quinidine), psychotropic medications antibiotics, for example, (cotrimoxazole, ciprofloxacin, levofloxacin, gatifloxacin, and moxifloxacin). In addition, Clarithromycin has also been implicated in many hypoglycemia cases, and the risk of hypoglycemia is exceptionally high in the concomitant use of repaglinide [3, 11, 13]. A systematic review conducted in 2008 and included 448 references assessed 164 drugs associated with hypoglycemia [14], the most commonly mentioned drugs to be linked with hypoglycemia were—quinolones, pentamidine, quinine, beta-blockers, angiotensin-converting enzyme inhibitors (ACEI), and IGF.

2.1.2 Insulin-related causes

2.1.2.1 Absolute insulin excess

Both absolute and relative insulin excess is a major cause of hypoglycemia. Absolute insulin excess occurs due to excessive insulin doses, wrong time of injection, wrong insulin type, and decreased insulin clearance as in renal failure and ill-timed.

Therefore, the antidiabetic regimen should be adjusted according to a review of blood glucose patterns. In addition, understanding the pharmacokinetic profile of different types of insulin is a key to dosing insulin safely [6, 8, 10, 15].

2.1.2.2 Relative insulin excess

The relative insulin excess occurs due to:

a. Decreased exogenous glucose delivery

The risk of hypoglycemia is increased during overnight fasting and with exercise. A new exercise routine, duration, intensity, and inadequate energy intake can increase insulin sensitivity and glucose utilization. The glucose utilization/insulin dose mismatch can increase the risk of hypoglycemia. It is worth mentioning that insulin doses on days of planned exercise should be well-controlled. Patients need to associate the meal with inulin injection and need to understand how the carbohydrates in their diet affect blood glucose [9, 12, 16]. Inherently, delayed meals, inadequate carbohydrate intake, and skipping meals or snacks can increase the risk of hypoglycemia [17].

b. Increased insulin sensitivity

The body's insulin sensitivity following weight loss or improved glycemic control often increases during midnight [6, 8].

c. Decreased endogenous glucose production

The effects of alcohol on blood glucose levels depend on the amount of alcohol consumption and the fed status of the individual. Acute alcohol intake after a fasting state (3–4 days) can induce severe hypoglycemia even in a healthy individual. Alcohol intake has an inhibitory effect on gluconeogenesis [13].

2.1.3 Diabetic complications (gastroparesis, neuropathy)

Gastroparesis, that is, delayed gastric emptying, is common autonomic neuropathy in patients with long-standing diabetes. It results in poor glycemic control and poor nutrition, and dehydration, resulting in frequent hypoglycemia episodes, hospitalizations, and poor quality of life [18, 19]. Neuropathy is also associated with hypoglycemia, particularly hypoglycemia-associated autonomic failure (HAAF). HAAF is a situation in which there is an absence or reduction of insulin secretion, enhancement of glucagon secretion, and/or a defective glucose counter-regulation by epinephrine. These factors induce hypoglycemia by reducing sympathetic neural activity and neurogenic symptoms [20].

2.1.4 Malabsorption (Celiac disease, pancreatic exocrine insufficiency)

Celiac disease is a chronic autoimmune disorder that destructs the small intestine, so the patient is unable to take nutrients in. It is prevalent in type 1 diabetes and causes episodes of hypoglycemia. Pancreatic exocrine insufficiency, which is characterized by a deficiency of exocrine pancreatic enzymes, is also associated with type I and II diabetes.

2.1.5 Hormone deficiency (cortisol, growth hormone, hypopituitarism, glucagon, and epinephrine deficiency in insulin-deficient diabetes)

The hormonal deficiency was found to be associated with hypoglycemia. Cortisol and growth hormone deficiencies, for instance, cause a reduction in gluconeogenesis and increased glucose utilization leading to hypoglycemia. Moreover, isolated glucagon deficiency can also result in hypoglycemia if insulin secretion is not suppressed and the counter-regulatory hormone epinephrine secretion is decreased. Studies also found that hypopituitarism may present with life-threatening hypoglycemia [21].

2.1.6 Concurrent illness (renal, hepatic, or cardiac failure, sepsis)

Hypoglycemia developing secondary to an underlying illness is associated with increased nutritional body demand due to increased metabolic response in critically ill patients. Endogenous glucose production is rapidly reduced in hepatic diseases and liver cirrhosis [22].

As kidneys play a major role in metabolizing insulin, reabsorption and synthesizing glucose, and excretion of different metabolites of hypoglycemic medications. Therefore, kidney impairment will prohibit all these processes leading to hypoglycemia. On the other hand, the counter-regulatory response to hypoglycemia may be defective due to uremia and associated anorexia [21]. On the other hand, in uremia, gluconeogenesis from the kidney and liver is reduced. Hypoglycemia can also occur in acute renal failure and end-stage renal disease (ESR), this is due to reduced renal insulinase-mediated insulin clearance.

Furthermore, severe cardiac failure and hepatic congestion may contribute to lower glucose output from the liver and reduce its intestinal absorption. While hypoglycemia in sepsis and adrenal insufficiency develops due to increased serum cortisol levels [4]. In literature, hypoglycemia in sepsis is often related to strict glycemic control protocols for stress hyperglycemia [23–27].

2.1.7 Psychological

2.1.7.1 Fear of hypoglycemia

The fear of hypoglycemia is common in patients with diabetes. It influences the quality and health outcomes. It can also increase the risk of poor metabolic control [28].

2.1.7.2 Depression

In diabetic patients with depression, hypoglycemia can occur frequently as a result of poor adherence to medications, diet, physical activity, smoking cessation, poor self-care, and blood glucose monitoring [29].

2.1.7.3 Cognitive impairment

Cognitive dysfunction and dementia may increase the risk of hypoglycemia, especially in elderly patients [30]. Although the association remains unclear, it is thought that person with cognitive disabilities will have errors in taking his medication [21].

3. Non-diabetic hypoglycemia

3.1 Non-diabetic hypoglycemia: overview

Non-diabetic hypoglycemia (hypoglycemia without diabetes) is a rare condition, it comes from having too much insulin in the blood, leading to low blood glucose levels. It can occur in pre-diabetes, sepsis, and critical organ failure including renal or hepatic failure. It also rarely occurs in cortisol deficiency [8], and β-cell tumors due to endogenous hyperinsulinism [8, 31–33]. Moreover, hypoglycemia can be accidental, surreptitious, or even malicious [34].

Hypoglycemia can occur post-bariatric surgery, that is, gastric bypass surgery, or even due to an autoimmune disease [8, 32, 33]. **Table 2** demonstrates the causes of hypoglycemia in nondiabetic patients.

3.2 Differential diagnosis

Whipple's triad (low plasma glucose level, clinical signs or symptoms of hypoglycemia, and resolution of signs or symptoms when the plasma glucose level increases) should be documented prior to initiating an evaluation [35].

When the patient is either looking ill or medicated, the initial diagnosis should focus on the possibility of drug involvement, critical conditions, hormone deficiency, or non-islet cell tumor hypoglycemia. If the patient seems well in the absence of any of the fore-mentioned etiologies, the focus should be on the possibility of having endogenous hyperinsulinism due to insulinomas, functional β-cell disorders, or insulin autoimmune conditions. In addition to the possibility of accidental, surreptitious,

Drugs Salicylates Sulfa drug antibiotics Pentamidine Quinine	Hormone deficiency Cortisol Growth hormone Glucagon Epinephrine Hypopituitarism
Critical illness Renal failure Hepatic failure Cardiac failure Sepsis Inanition	Endogenous hyperinsulinism Insulinoma Nesidioblastosis Post-gastric bypass surgery
Non-islet cell tumor	Insulin autoimmune hypoglycemia Antibody to insulin Antibody to the insulin receptor
Intentional/accidental Surreptitious Malicious Factitious	Infancy and childhood Preterm Infants of DM mother Maternal drugs-sulphonylureas Rh incompatibility Beckwith-Wiedemann syndrome Exchange transfusions Enzyme defects-glycogen storage the disease I, III, VI.

Table 2.
Causes of hypoglycemia in nondiabetic patients.

or malicious hypoglycemia [35, 36]. Hypoglycemia in patients post-bariatric surgery is increasingly recognized as the frequency of these operations has grown in the last few decades [36].

3.3 Etiology

3.3.1 Drug-induced

Fasting hypoglycemia is found to be associated with several medications, such as salicylates pain killers, antibiotic sulfa drugs, pentamidine, and quinine antimalarial medications [1].

3.3.2 Critical illnesses

Dysglycemia, in the form of hyperglycemia, hypoglycemia, and/or marked glucose variability, is a characteristic feature of critical illness in both diabetic and non-diabetic patients [37]. It can increase morbidity and mortality [38]. Among hospitalized patients, serious illnesses, such as renal, hepatic, or cardiac failure; sepsis; and inanition are the only drugs to cause hypoglycemia.

3.3.2.1 Sepsis

Sepsis is one of the main causes of death across the world and is considered the most familiar cause of death among intensive care unit (ICU) patients [39]. The mortality rate due to sepsis ranges from 15 to 56% [40]. Not to mention that patients with sepsis usually report variable types of dysglycemia due to the changes in endocrine metabolism in sepsis, which affects the stability of the internal environment and worsens their general condition [41].

Sepsis patients are often complicated by hypoglycemia as has been approved by multiple large-scale randomized controlled trials (RCTs). Although such protocols have not been approved to improve patient mortality, rather they possibly increase the risk of hypoglycemia [41]. While there is a dearth of studies on the effects of spontaneous hypoglycemia in patients with sepsis, its occurrence leads to increased mortality and elevated lactate levels in patients with sepsis [41].

In septic patients, increased glucose utilization is induced by cytokine production in macrophage-rich tissues, such as the liver, spleen, and lung. Hypoglycemia develops if glucose production fails to keep pace. Cytokine-induced inhibition of gluconeogenesis in the setting of nutritional glycogen depletion, in combination with hepatic and renal hypoperfusion, may also contribute to hypoglycemia.

3.3.2.2 Hepatic failure

The liver as a metabolic organ plays an important role in glucose metabolism. It regulates the blood glucose level mainly through glycogenolysis and gluconeogenesis. Hepatic impairment is well known to correlate with poor blood glucose regulation [42]. The presence of liver impairment or hepatocellular damage can lead to a disturbance of the metabolic function of the liver causing an imbalance in blood glucose levels. Rapid and extensive hepatic destruction, such as toxic hepatitis, for example, causes fasting hypoglycemia due to the lack of endogenous glucose production.

3.3.2.3 Renal failure

Patients with end-stage kidney disease frequently experience variable glycemic disturbances, with the common incidence of both hypoglycemia and hyperglycemia. The risk of hypoglycemia is increased in critically ill renal patients and having chronic kidney disease is a known risk factor for developing hypoglycemia [43, 44]. Multiple mechanisms are involved in hypoglycemia development in kidney disease patients, including impaired gluconeogenesis process run by the kidney, impaired insulin clearance by the kidney, and impaired insulin degradation due to uremia.

Other mechanisms of developing hypoglycemia in kidney disease also include increased erythrocyte glucose uptake during hemodialysis, impaired counter-regulatory hormone responses (cortisol, growth hormone), and nutritional deprivation [45–49]. Moreover, insulin sensitivity may improve in uremic patients after starting renal replacement therapy increases the risk of hypoglycemia in renal replacement patients [50]. In contrast, the risk of hypoglycemia is reduced with starting hemodialysis due to the addition of glucose to the dialysis solution [51].

3.3.2.4 Cardiac failure

Severe heart failure is sometimes associated with hypoglycemia. However, the exact mechanism is yet to be determined. Several mechanisms have been suggested including impaired gluconeogenesis due to hepatic congestion and the reduced glycogen stores from either inadequate intake or reduced gastrointestinal absorption [52–54].

3.3.2.5 Inanition

Inanition is a well-known cause of hypoglycemia. During starvation, a catabolic state occurs when the body shifts from predominately carbohydrate metabolism to that of fat and protein, the brain then starts conversing and utilizing alternative substrates, such as lactate, pyruvate, and ketone bodies with only a modest counter-regulatory neuroendocrine and autonomic nervous system response.

The refeeding syndrome (RFS) can occur after starvation and energy replenishment. This can be defined as severe electrolyte and metabolic abnormalities in undernourished patients after the introduction of nutrients [55–57]. Multiple organ systems including cardiac, respiratory, neurologic, and hematologic can be affected by the RFS and are occasionally associated with postprandial hypoglycemia [55, 58].

3.3.3 Hormone deficiencies

Increased cortisol and growth hormone (GH) secretion are involved in the defense mechanism against prolonged hypoglycemia. When these defenses fail to refute the hypoglycemia episode, plasma glucose levels will continue to fall [35].

Chronic cortisol deficiency is typically associated with anorexia and weight loss, likely leading to glycogen depletion. Cortisol deficiency is also associated with impaired gluconeogenesis and low levels of gluconeogenic precursors causing the substrate limited gluconeogenesis, in the setting of glycogen depletion, which leads to hypoglycemia.

Growth hormone deficiency can cause hypoglycemia in young children. In addition to extended fasting, high rates of glucose utilization, such as during exercise and in pregnancy, or low rates of glucose production, such as post-alcohol consumption, can precipitate hypoglycemia in adults with previously undiagnosed hypopituitarism [59].

3.3.4 Non-islet cell tumor hypoglycemia (NICTH)

Hypoglycemia due to non-islet cell tumors abbreviated as NICTH is considered to be rare [8, 31–33]; it is a rare paraneoplastic syndrome encountered in the setting of a wide variety of tumors and is most common in tumors of mesenchymal or hepatic origin [60]. Hypoglycemia in this realm is initially attributed to glucose consumption by the tumor and to tumor secretion of an "insulin-like" factor afterward, this factor is a precursor of IGF-2, called Big-IGF-2. While secretion of Big-IGF2 is the most common cause of NICTH, secretion of somatostatin or IGF1 may also be responsible [61]. Usually, IGF-2-related hypoglycemia manifests when the tumor turns quite large [62, 63].

3.3.5 Endogenous hyperinsulinism

Endogenous hyperinsulinism is a clinical condition that involves excessive insulin secretion and is related in 55% of cases to insulinoma [64]. Nesidioblastosis and insulinoma represent the main cause of endogenous hyperinsulinemic hypoglycemia in infants and apparently healthy adults, respectively [35]. The main pathophysiological feature of endogenous hyperinsulinism is the failure of insulin secretion to fall to very low levels when plasma glucose concentrations fall to hypoglycemic levels; hypoglycemia in this case is a result of low rates of glucose production, rather than high rates of glucose utilization [65]. Nesidioblastosis is a rare cause of persistent hyperinsulinemic hypoglycemia in adults. The hypoglycemia in the case of nesidioblastosis is attributed to β-cell hypertrophy and hyperfunction [66–68].

Post-prandial hypoglycemia can also be observed after bariatric surgeries, especially the procedures that divert nutrients into the mid-small bowel, such as Roux-en-Y gastric bypass surgery (RYGB), and not fully restrictive procedures like adjustable gastric banding [69]. Post-RYGB surgery hypoglycemia (PGBH) usually occurs between 1 and 8 years after the procedure [70], this might be due to several causes including late dumping syndrome, nesidioblastosis, and insulinoma [71].

3.3.6 Insulin autoimmune hypoglycemia

Hypoglycemia can also be caused by an antibody to insulin or its receptors, a condition known as insulin autoimmune syndrome (IAS) and also known as Hirata's disease or insulin autoimmune hypoglycemia (IAH). It is essentially a rare autoimmune disorder caused by the spontaneous production of anti-insulin and anti-insulin receptor antibodies which bind insulin/proinsulin and/or insulin receptors and work as insulin-mimetic leading to predominantly postprandial hyperinsulinemic hypoglycemia [9, 72]. Graves' disease is frequently present in Hirata syndrome and appears to be particularly prevalent in Japan [73].

3.3.7 Intentional/accidental

Hypoglycemia can also happen accidentally and can be surreptitious, malicious, or sometimes fictitious [74]. Pharmacy errors (e.g., substitution of a hypoglycemic drug for another medication) and medical treatment errors can stand behind some accidental intake cases [75].

Intentional hypoglycemia can be surreptitious and this is most commonly seen in people with knowledge of and access to glucose-lowering medications. It can be malicious which is usually accomplished by the administration of insulin or an insulin secretagogue [74]. It also can be fictitious in some cases.

3.3.8 Infancy and childhood

Hyperinsulinemic hypoglycemia (HH), which is characterized by unregulated insulin release, is the most common cause of persistent and severe hypoglycemia in infants and children [76]. This can be transient (associated with risk factors), or permanent (linked to genetic mutations). In the majority of cases (60–70%) hypoglycemia occurs in the first week of life [77, 78], and it carries a considerable risk of neurological damage and developmental delays if diagnosis and treatment were delayed [76].

HH is also classified as primary and secondary HH. The primary HH, which is also known as congenital HH (CHH), where the hypoglycemia is associated with variants in several genes involved in pancreatic development and function. The secondary HH, where hypoglycemia is associated with syndromes, such as intrauterine growth restriction, maternal diabetes, and birth asphyxia [79].

CHI can be classified according to etiology into two types—acquired and genetic. In neonates, acquired forms are usually associated with some conditions, such as perinatal stress or maternal gestational diabetes, and are often transient [80]. Genetic CHI can be caused by single-gene mutations in the insulin secretory pathway or genes causing syndromes with multiple associated factors, such as Beckwith-Wiedemann syndrome or Kabuki syndrome [78].

Hypoglycemia in infants can also be caused by counter-regulatory hormone deficiencies, such as adrenal insufficiency or GH deficiency [80]. In such cases, replacement of the deficient hormones yields a complete resolution of hypoglycemia. Some metabolic disorders, such as fatty acid oxidation disorders and certain glycogen storage disease types, are additional causes of hypoglycemia in infants and children [81].

DOI: http://dx.doi.org/10.5772/intechopen.105061

Author details

Ala' Abu-Odeh*, Dalal Alnatour and Leen Fino
Applied Science Private University, Amman, Jordan

*Address all correspondence to: a_abuodeh@asu.edu.jo

References

[1] Desimone ME, Weinstock RS. Non-diabetic hypoglycemia. The Journal of Clinical Endocrinology and Metabolism. 2016;**98**(10):39A

[2] Seaquist ER, Anderson J, Childs B, Cryer P, Dagogo-Jack S, Fish L, et al. Hypoglycemia and diabetes: A report of a workgroup of the American Diabetes Association and the Endocrine Society. The Journal of Clinical Endocrinology and Metabolism. 2013;**98**(5):1845-1859

[3] Kalra S, Mukherjee JJ, Venkataraman S, Bantwal G, Shaikh S, Saboo B, et al. Hypoglycemia: The neglected complication. Indian Journal of Endocrinology and Metabolism. 2013;**17**(5):819

[4] Toor A, Toor A, Krishnamurthy M. Critical illness associated fatal hypoglycemia in a nondiabetic male. Case Reports in Critical Care. USA 2019;**2019**:1-3

[5] Cryer PE. Hypoglycemia. In: Endocrine Emergencies. USA: Springer; 2021. pp. 27-35

[6] Oyer DS. The science of hypoglycemia in patients with diabetes. Current Diabetes Reviews. 2013;**9**(3):195-208

[7] Cryer PE, Axelrod L, Grossman AB, Heller SR, Montori VM, Seaquist ER, et al. Evaluation and management of adult hypoglycemic disorders: An Endocrine Society Clinical Practice Guideline. The Journal of Clinical Endocrinology and Metabolism. Elsevier, Amsterdam 2009;**94**(3):709-728

[8] Cryer PE, Polonsky K. Glucose homeostasis and hypoglycemia. In: Williams Textbook of Endocrinology. Vol. 88. Amsterdam: Elsevier; 2008. pp. 1589-1590

[9] Douillard C, Jannin A, Vantyghem MC. Rare causes of hypoglycemia in adults. 2020 [2213-3941 (Electronic)]

[10] Evans Kreider K, Pereira K, Padilla BI. Practical approaches to diagnosing, treating and preventing hypoglycemia in diabetes. Diabetes Therapy. 2017;**8**(6):1427-1435

[11] Murad MH, Coto-Yglesias F, Wang AT, Sheidaee N, Mullan RJ, Elamin MB, et al. Drug-induced hypoglycemia: A systematic review. The Journal of Clinical Endocrinology and Metabolism. 2009;**94**(3):741-745

[12] Lamounier RN, Geloneze B, Leite SO, Montenegro R, Zajdenverg L, Fernandes M, et al. Hypoglycemia incidence and awareness among insulin-treated patients with diabetes: The HAT study in Brazil. Diabetology and Metabolic Syndrome. 2018;**10**(1):1-10

[13] Kalaria T, Ko YL, Issuree KKJ. Literature review: Drug and alcohol-induced hypoglycaemia. Journal of Laboratory and Precision Medicine. 2021:1-16

[14] Murad MH, Coto-Yglesias F, Wang AT, Sheidaee N, Mullan RJ, Elamin MB, Erwin PJ, et al. Clinical review: Drug-induced hypoglycemia: A systematic review [1945-7197 (Electronic)], USA

[15] Vanek C, Loriaux L. Endocrine Emergencies: Recognition and Treatment. USA: Springer; 2021

[16] Cryer P. Hypoglycemia in Diabetes: Pathophysiology, Prevalence, and Prevention. USA: American Diabetes Association; 2016

[17] Silbert R, Salcido-Montenegro A, Rodriguez-Gutierrez R, Katabi A, McCoy RG. Hypoglycemia among patients with type 2 diabetes: Epidemiology, risk factors, and prevention strategies. Current Diabetes Reports. 2018;**18**(8):1-16

[18] Krishnasamy S, Abell TL. Diabetic gastroparesis: Principles and current trends in management. Diabetes Therapy. 2018;**9**(1):1-42

[19] Homko C, Siraj ES, Parkman HP. The impact of gastroparesis on diabetes control: Patient perceptions. Journal of Diabetes and its Complications. 2016;**30**(5):826-829

[20] Yanai H, Adachi H, Katsuyama H, Moriyama S, Hamasaki H, Sako A. Causative anti-diabetic drugs and the underlying clinical factors for hypoglycemia in patients with diabetes. World Journal of Diabetes. 2015;**6**(1):30

[21] Martín-Timón I, del Cañizo-Gómez FJ. Mechanisms of hypoglycemia unawareness and implications in diabetic patients. World Journal of Diabetes. 2015;**6**(7):912

[22] Narla RR, Hashimoto T, Kelly K, Heaney A. Hypoglycemia: A tale of three causes. Journal of Clinical and Translational Endocrinology: Case Reports. 2016;**2**:4-6

[23] Metzger S, Nusair S, Planer D, Barash V, Pappo O, Shilyansky J, et al. Inhibition of hepatic gluconeogenesis and enhanced glucose uptake contribute to the development of hypoglycemia in mice bearing interleukin-1β-secreting tumor. Endocrinology. 2004;**145**(11):5150-5156

[24] Brunkhorst FM, Engel C, Bloos F, Meier-Hellmann A, Ragaller M, Weiler N, et al. Intensive insulin therapy and pentastarch resuscitation in severe sepsis. New England Journal of Medicine. 2008;**358**(2):125-139

[25] Kalfon P, Giraudeau B, Ichai C, Guerrini A, Brechot N, Cinotti R, et al. Tight computerized versus conventional glucose control in the ICU: A randomized controlled trial. Intensive Care Medicine. 2014;**40**(2):171-181

[26] Tanner O. Intensive versus conventional glucose control in critically ill patients. New England Journal of Medicine. 2009;**360**(13):1283-1297

[27] Maitra SR, Wojnar MM, Lang CH. Alterations in tissue glucose uptake during the hyperglycemic and hypoglycemic phases of sepsis. Shock. 2000;**13**(5):379-385

[28] Anderbro T, Gonder-Frederick L, Bolinder J, Lins P-E, Wredling R, Moberg E, et al. Fear of hypoglycemia: Relationship to hypoglycemic risk and psychological factors. Acta Diabetologica. 2015;**52**(3):581-589

[29] Katon WJ, Young BA, Russo J, Lin EH, Ciechanowski P, Ludman EJ, et al. Association of depression with increased risk of severe hypoglycemic episodes in patients with diabetes. Annals of Family Medicine. 2013;**11**(3):245-250

[30] Yun J-S, Ko S-H. Risk factors and adverse outcomes of severe hypoglycemia in type 2 diabetes mellitus. Diabetes and Metabolism Journal. 2016;**40**(6):423-432

[31] Service F. Hypoglycemic disorders. New England Journal of Medicine. 1995;**332**(17):1144-1152

[32] Service FJ. Classification of hypoglycemic disorders. Endocrinology and Metabolism Clinics of North America. 1999;**28**(3):501-517

[33] Guettier J-M, Gorden P. Hypoglycemia. Endocrinology and Metabolism Clinics. 2006;**35**(4):753-766

[34] Marks V, Teale JD. Drug-induced hypoglycemia. Endocrinology and Metabolism Clinics. 1999;**28**(3):555-577

[35] Cryer PE, Axelrod L, Grossman AB, Heller SR, Montori VM, Seaquist ER, Service FJ, et al. Evaluation and management of adult hypoglycemic disorders: An Endocrine Society Clinical Practice Guideline [1945-7197 (Electronic)]

[36] Madunić J, Madunić IV, Gajski G, Popić J, Garaj-Vrhovac V. Apigenin: A dietary flavonoid with diverse anticancer properties. Cancer Letters. 2018;**413**:11-22

[37] Van den Berghe G. How does blood glucose control with insulin save lives in intensive care? [0021-9738 (Print)]

[38] Pérez-Calatayud ÁA, Guillén-Vidaña A, Fraire-Félix IS, Anica-Malagón ED, Briones Garduño JC, Carrillo-Esper R. Metabolic control in the critically ill patient an update: Hyperglycemia, glucose variability hypoglycemia and relative hypoglycemia [2444-054X (Electronic)]

[39] Fleischmann C, Scherag A, Adhikari NK, Hartog CS, Tsaganos T, Schlattmann P, et al. Assessment of global incidence and mortality of hospital-treated sepsis. Current Estimates and Limitations [1535-4970 (Electronic)]

[40] Bauer M, Gerlach H, Vogelmann T, Preissing F, Stiefel J, Adam D. Mortality in sepsis and septic shock in Europe, North America and Australia between 2009 and 2019—Results from a systematic review and meta-analysis. Critical Care. 2020;**24**(1):239

[41] Wang J, Zhu CK, Yu JQ, Tan R, Yang PL. Hypoglycemia and mortality in sepsis patients: A systematic review and meta-analysis [1527-3288 (Electronic)]

[42] Kumar R. Hepatogenous diabetes: An underestimated problem of liver cirrhosis [2230-8210 (Print)]

[43] Fischer KF, Lees JA, Newman JH. Hypoglycemia in hospitalized patients. Causes and Outcomes [0028-4793 (Print)]

[44] Arem R. Hypoglycemia associated with renal failure [0889-8529 (Print)]

[45] Sobngwi E, Enoru S, Ashuntantang G, Azabji-Kenfack M, Dehayem M, Onana A, et al. Day-to-day variation of insulin requirements of patients with type 2 diabetes and end-stage renal disease undergoing maintenance hemodialysis. Diabetes Care. 2010;**33**(7):1409-1412

[46] Rahhal M-N, Gharaibeh NE, Rahimi L, Ismail-Beigi F. Disturbances in insulin-glucose metabolism in patients with advanced renal disease with and without diabetes. The Journal of Clinical Endocrinology and Metabolism. 2019;**104**(11):4949-4966

[47] Gianchandani RY, Neupane S, Iyengar JJ, Heung M. Pathophysiology and management of hypoglycemiain end-stage renal disease patients: A review. Endocrine Practice. 2017;**23**(3):353-362

[48] Mak RH, De Fronzo RA. Glucose and insulin metabolism in uremia. Nephron. 1992;**61**(4):377-382

[49] Tuttle KR, Bakris GL, Bilous RW, Chiang JL, De Boer IH, Goldstein-Fuchs J, et al. Diabetic kidney disease: A report from an ADA Consensus Conference. Diabetes Care. 2014;**37**(10):2864-2883

[50] DeFronzo RA, Tobin JD, Rowe JW, Andres R. Glucose intolerance in uremia. Quantification of pancreatic beta cell sensitivity to glucose and tissue sensitivity to insulin [0021-9738 (Print)]

[51] Burmeister JE, Scapini A, da Rosa Miltersteiner D, da Costa MG, Campos BM. Glucose-added dialysis fluid prevents asymptomatic hypoglycaemia in regular haemodialysis [0931-0509 (Print)]

[52] Kittah NE, Vella A. Management of endocrine disease: Pathogenesis and management of hypoglycemia [1479-683X (Electronic)]

[53] Sako A, Yasunaga H, Matsui H, Fushimi K, Hamasaki H, Katsuyama H, Tsujimoto T, et al. Hospitalization with hypoglycemia in patients without diabetes mellitus: A retrospective study using a national inpatient database in Japan. 2008-2012 [1536-5964 (Electronic)]

[54] Mellinkoff SM, Tumulty PA. Hepatic hypoglycemia; its occurrence in congestive heart failure [0028-4793 (Print)]

[55] Boateng AA, Sriram K, Meguid MM, Crook M. Refeeding syndrome: Treatment considerations based on collective analysis of literature case reports [1873-1244 (Electronic)]

[56] Solomon SM, Kirby DF. The refeeding syndrome: A review [0148-6071 (Print)]

[57] Crook MA, Hally V, Panteli JV. The importance of the refeeding syndrome [0899-9007 (Print)]

[58] Heruc GA, Little TJ, Kohn MR, Madden S, Clarke SD, Horowitz M, et al. Effects of starvation and short-term refeeding on gastric emptying and postprandial blood glucose regulation in adolescent girls with anorexia nervosa [1522-1555 (Electronic)]

[59] Reznik Y, Barat P, Bertherat J, Bouvattier C, Castinetti F, Chabre O, et al. SFE/SFEDP adrenal insufficiency French consensus: Introduction and handbook [Consensus sur l'insuffisance surrénale de la SFE/SFEDP: introduction et guide]. Annales d'Endocrinologie. 2018;**79**(1):1-22

[60] Teale JD, Marks V. Glucocorticoid therapy suppresses abnormal secretion of big IGF-II by non-islet cell tumours inducing hypoglycaemia (NICTH). Clinical Endocrinology. 1998;**49**(4):491-498

[61] Daughaday WH. Hypoglycemia due to paraneoplastic secretion of insulin-like growth factor-I. The Journal of Clinical Endocrinology and Metabolism. 2007;**92**(5):1616

[62] Phillips LS, Robertson DG. Insulin-like growth factors and non-islet cell tumor hypoglycemia. Metabolism. 1993;**42**(9):1093-1101

[63] Dynkevich Y, Rother KI, Whitford I, Qureshi S, Galiveeti S, Szulc AL, et al. Tumors, IGF-2, and hypoglycemia: Insights from the clinic, the laboratory, and the historical archive. Endocrine Reviews. 2013;**34**(6):798-826

[64] Phan GQ, Yeo CJ, Hruban RH, Littemoe KD, Pitt HA, Cameron JL. Surgical experience with pancreatic and peripancreatic neuroendocrine tumors: Review of 125 patients. Journal of Gastrointestinal Surgery. 1998;**2**(5):473-482

[65] Rizza RA, Haymond MW, Verdonk CA, Mandarino LJ, Miles JM, Service FJ, et al. Pathogenesis of hypoglycemia in insulinoma patients: Suppression of

hepatic glucose production by insulin. Diabetes. 1981;**30**(5):377-381

[66] Dravecka I, Lazurova I. Nesidioblastosis in adults. Neoplasma. 2014;**61**(3):252-256

[67] Jabri A, Bayard C. Nesidioblastosis associated with hyperinsulinemic hypoglycemia in adults: Review of the literature. European Journal of Internal Medicine. 2004;**15**(7):407-410

[68] Anlauf M, Wieben D, Perren A, Sipos B, Komminoth P, Raffel A, et al. Persistenthyperinsulinemichypoglycemia in 15 adults with diffuse nesidioblastosis: Diagnostic criteria, incidence, and characterization of β-cell changes. The American Journal of Surgical Pathology. 2005;**29**(4):524-533

[69] Salehi M, Vella A, McLaughlin T, Patti ME. Hypoglycemia after gastric bypass surgery: Current concepts and controversies. The Journal of Clinical Endocrinology and Metabolism. 2018;**103**(8):2815-2826

[70] Service GJ, Thompson GB, Service FJ, Andrews JC, Collazo-Clavell ML, Lloyd RV. Hyperinsulinemic hypoglycemia with nesidioblastosis after gastric-bypass surgery. The New England Journal of Medicine. 2005;**353**(3):249-254

[71] Moreira RO, Moreira RB, Machado NA, Gonçalves TB, Coutinho WF. Post-prandial hypoglycemia after bariatric surgery: Pharmacological treatment with verapamil and acarbose. Obesity Surgery. 2008;**18**(12):1618-1621

[72] Ismail AA. The insulin autoimmune syndrome (IAS) as a cause of hypoglycaemia: An update on the pathophysiology, biochemical investigations and diagnosis. Clinical Chemistry and Laboratory Medicine. 2016;**54**(11):1715-1724

[73] Paudyal B, Shakya M, Basnyat B. Spontaneous hypoglycaemia in a patient with Graves' disease. BMJ Case Reports 2016;2016:bcr2016214801

[74] Marks V, Teale JD. Hypoglycemia: Factitious and felonious. Endocrinology and Metabolism Clinics of North America. 1999;**28**(3):579-601

[75] Bates DW. Unexpected hypoglycemia in a critically ill patient. Annals of Internal Medicine. 2002;**137**(2):110-116

[76] Banerjee I, Raskin J, Arnoux JB, De Leon DD, Weinzimer SA, Hammer M, et al. Congenital hyperinsulinism in infancy and childhood: Challenges, unmet needs and the perspective of patients and families. Orphanet Journal of Rare Diseases. 2022;**17**(1):61

[77] Arnoux J-B, Verkarre V, Saint-Martin C, Montravers F, Brassier A, Valayannopoulos V, et al. Congenital hyperinsulinism: Current trends in diagnosis and therapy. Orphanet Journal of Rare Diseases. 2011;**6**(1):63

[78] Banerjee I, Salomon-Estebanez M, Shah P, Nicholson J, Cosgrove KE, Dunne MJ. Therapies and outcomes of congenital hyperinsulinism-induced hypoglycaemia. Diabetic Medicine. 2019;**36**(1):9-21

[79] Güemes M, Rahman SA, Kapoor RR, Flanagan S, Houghton JAL, Misra S, et al. Hyperinsulinemic hypoglycemia in children and adolescents: Recent advances in understanding of pathophysiology and management. Reviews in Endocrine & Metabolic Disorders. 2020;**21**(4):577-597

[80] Halaby LP, Steinkrauss L. Hypoglycemia: Symptom or diagnosis?

Journal of Pediatric Nursing. 2012;**27**(1):97-99

[81] Thornton PS, Stanley CA, De Leon DD, Harris D, Haymond MW, Hussain K, et al. Recommendations from the Pediatric Endocrine Society for Evaluation and Management of Persistent Hypoglycemia in Neonates, Infants, and Children. The Journal of Pediatrics. 2015;**167**(2):238-245

Section 3

Diagnosis and Treatment of Hypoglycemia

Chapter 4

Blood Glucose Monitoring

Anujka Selea Zivojinovic

Abstract

Glucose monitoring is the integral part of diabetes management. We have over the years moved from qualifying sugars in urine to identifying glucose alone in the interstitial tissue. Even more we are anow able to identify and use minute to minuet glucose fluctuations and use them to avoid the dangers and unpleasantries of hypoglycemia. We look at the development of glucose monitoring methods. The development of classic basic glucose monitors as well as the development of continuous glucose monitors. Basic principles of function, advantages, and disadvantages, as well as areas of actual and projected use are mentioned. We name some of the patient groups that have proven to get most advantage of glucose monitoring. He need for individual approach an patient activation as well as for alert diabetes health care provided is necessary for optimal use of technology for glucose monitoring.

Keywords: glucose, glucose monitor, continuous glucose monitoring (CGM), intensified insulin treatment, hypoglycemia

1. Introduction

Diabetes mellitus is group of metabolic diseases, resulting from absent or defective insulin secretion and/or action and manifested by high blood glucose levels. We think of diabetes as of a chronic long and progressive disease that requires a complex multifaceted treatment.

At the time of insulin discovery, identification, and quantification of glucose was a demanding laboratory task. Today, glucose in blood is the most frequently analyzed parameter in a clinical chemistry laboratory. The value of global blood glucose monitoring systems market size in 2021. in the US was estimated at 14.78 billion dollars and with a projected to grow to over 31 billion dollars by 2029.

While it was the discovery of insulin, 100 years ago, that most profoundly shifted the perspective of diabetes form a lethal, relatively quickly progressive disease to a chronic progressive disease which increases risk for micro- and/or macrovascular complications, it was the availability of simple, easy to use, reliable glucose testing that has made diabetes, with its acute and chronic events (mostly hyperglycemia but also hypoglycemia), closer to every patient and living with diabetes more predictable. Glucose monitoring has, together with development of diabetes education programs, contributed to aiming the complex diabetes patient at being a "patient centered care" where "... patient values guide all clinical decisions".

It is the development of glucose monitoring systems that has made the health care providers and researchers focus again to the fact that glucose control is a continuum- diabetes with glucose swings and inappropriate glucose control is a disease of deviant homeostasis, where insulin plays the main, but not the only role. It may be that our approach to hyperglycemia and hypoglycemia will be changed in future, again, due to the observations got through glucose monitoring systems and our interventions.

The way to modern glucose monitoring equipment was not short and was not easy.

It was necessary with development of basal natural sciences to get form the intuitive to the quantitative and beyond...

1.1 The glucose molecule

The first glucose molecule was isolated from raisins in 1747 by Andreaas Marggraf. The name (glycos- sweet) was established and used in 1838 by Jean Baptiste Dumas.

Glucose is classified as a monosaccharide- simple sugar. The molecular formula C6H12 O2.

Glucose qualifies as a hexose, because it contains 6 carbon atoms. It an aldose- meaning that it contains an aldehyde group that is easily oxidized [1].

Friederich August Kekule proposed also the name dextrose, being aware of the ability of glucose water solution to turn the plane of polarized light to the right. The metabolically active glucose is D (+) glucose.

In 1902 the Nobel Prize for chemistry was given to Emil Fisher who explained the cyclic structure of glucose: Biologically active glucose is mostly in cyclic structure.

A few chemical properties are of significance when defining glucose, but the most important is borne by the aldehyde group. That redox capacity can translate in a subset of reactions leading to formation of colored substrates or electrochemical reaction.

1.2 Glucose, laboratory identification

It was in 1838, that George Rees, a physician at Guy's Hospital, London, isolated sugar and in excess from blood of a diabetic patient [2].

Monitoring of glucose was at first done through monitoring of glucose in the urine. That was not an easy task and it was of little clinical significance: the finding of glucose in the urine signified advanced disease. Hypoglycemia could not be verified. The technique was complicated. The method was at most semiquantitative. Basis for use lies in the classical Fehling and Benedict reaction:

In 1848. The German chemist Herman Von Fehling developed a test that was able to differentiate reducing (sugars with aldehyde group) from nonreducing (sugars with keto group). Reducing sugar (such as glucose is) would be reducing a cuprous ion that than changes color and precipitates. The reaction requires a temperature of almost 60°C.

Stanley Benedict developed a modified copper reagent urine glucose test in 1908. The test uses the same principle as Fehling `s test but was easier to perform. The test was the basic glucose-monitoring test for almost 50 years. Urinary test based on Benedict reaction was introduced for home use in 1925. Test tube was given at the doctor's office, with the required reagents measured and dispensed by the physician. But it was basically the first test that the patients could use at home [3].

Benedict test, as a semiquantitative method, was a cornerstone of glucose monitoring in over 50 years and can be thought of the ground self-monitoring test.

In 1925, 26-year-old Danish botanist Detlev Muller discovered glucose oxidase [4]. The discovery was overshadowed by the work of Otto Warburg og Christian Walter who in 1932–1933 discovered glucose 6 phosphate dehydrogenase, the first discovered flavoenzyme. That the reaction produces color is of significance for further development of analytics. Warburg got, else, the Nobel prize for discovery of the nature and mode of action of respiratory enzyme).

Today's glucose monitoring techniques, quantitative, are mostly based on enzymatic reactions- glucose oxidase, hexokinase, or glucose dehydrogenase. The enzyme changes (oxidizes) glucose, and the transfer of electrons causes chromogenic reaction. The change in color is detected photometrically. The electron flow can also be measured electrochemically [5]. The methods are quantitative.

None of these methods, that we, regardless of many analytical problems, think of as an acceptable and reliable (also accurate and precise) reflection of blood glucose [6], would be in use had it not been for the basic chemical and physicochemical research done from the 1800.

2. Glucose monitoring: moving towards the patient

Benedict's reaction was developed in 1908. In 1925. we had a test for elf testing of glucose in the urine. It was a test that could be done home, but it was long from practical and it was necessary that the doctor gives the necessary equipment. In 1945, Ames (Elkhart, IN) developed a tablet with modified copper reagent, Clinitest. The method was also based on Benedicts reaction, but it was easier to perform. The method was semiquantitative and estimated the level of urinary glucose by comparison to the color chart.

By the late e1940 ies Hellen Fee (Mile's laboratories – which was known for producing Alca Selzer) developed the "dip and read" urine test – known as Clinistix. This was a huge step forward in clinical laboratory – the reagents for complete oxidative chain of reactions were set on a filter paper strip and could instantly identify glucose.

In 1957 Kohn showed that Clinistix could also give approximate results for blood glucose [7].

Dry chemistry came in to stay. In 1964, Boehringer Ingelheim introduced first Combur test that could identify glucose, protein, pH in the urine, and later Ketostix that could also identify ketones.

The first test strip for blood glucose was introduced in 1964: Ames -Mile's laboratories presented Dextrostix. Earnest C Adams was the developer. The test was based on glucose oxidase reaction. It included a semipermeable membrane that allowed glucose, but not the red blood cells to get to the reagent. The method was semiquantitative. It was meant for use at the doctor's office. The strips were widely used by the health care personnel at different points of health care, regardless that there were too many steps in the procedure ant too many steps that could lead to an inaccurate result. Stix limitations have been the trigger to develop automatic electronic glucose test strip reader, with standardized precision and quantitative results.

2.1 Glucose monitoring- glucometers come

Therefore, the first glucometer came. It was in 1970. It used Dextrostix. High cost, weight *at* 1,2 kg and only available at the doctor's office. Even the lighter and improved version produced by the Japanese in 1972, was a long way from what we think of as glucometer. It required repeated calibration, operator training and continuing practice, but with imminent insecurity about precision and variability.

It was developed further to a Glucometer 1, that came in 1981, as a first portable lightweight glucometer. It used again Dextrostix, and it was recommended for bedside monitoring of blood glucose. Glucometer 1 used a hexokinase-based glucose method.

In 1987. Came also the first blood glucose biosensor system. It used glucose oxidase strip. The electron transfer, stepwise, generated a current detected by amperometic sensor. It was the third generation of blood glucose monitoring systems. This was the final step that enabled the development of improved and easily used precise blood glucose monitoring instruments.

By the 1990 we have so moved from large instruments that required many analytical steps and the required blood volume for analysis was significantly reduced. Analytical time was reduced. High requirements for accuracy and precision are well met - while the first tests had variability of up to 40%, todays requirements today are less than 5% between meters and laboratory methods [8]. The development of software allows for keeping the measurements and eventually can make them available for analysis.

As much as chemistry and technology advanced, it is also the knowledge about diabetes that was pushing to test that would be reliable easy to use and available.

3. Continuous glucose monitoring (CGM): the principle

Continuous glucose measurement systems measure glucose in the interstitial fluid by a device that is inserted subcutaneously. The CGM system contains the sensor, a transmitter and a receiver or monitor.

The components have undergone significant changes from the first presented CGM system.

The first ever CGM system was approved by the FDA in 1999. It was produced by Medtronic (Medtronic guardian RT).

The device was measuring glucose in the interstitial fluid every 5 minutes. Glucose sensing electrode was inserted subcutaneously in the abdomen or in the arm. Glucose was measured electrochemically. The sensor lasted for 3 days. The results were stored and could be analyzed at the doctor's office. The data was not real time data ant the patient did not have access to data self. The patient could not get information about imminent hypoglycemia/hyperglycemia. The system needed calibration by fingerstick glucose measurements every 6–12 hours. The sensor and the receiver were physically connected by a cable that transmitted the measurements. The CGM could collect data in a three-day period [9]. Also, far away from the CGM systems that we know today.

The revolutionary, however, was that the glucose was measured often (1–5 minutes). The number of fingerstick was reduced – to calibration and eventually to check the results. The first generations of CGMS were basically only for professional use: the patients did not have insight into the glucose levels in the observation period. The first CGMs had an exceptionally large glucose variability, something that, naturally, was not wanted.

3.1 Continuous glucose monitoring (CGM): some important steps

The first real time CGM was the Glucowatch biographer (Cygnos, Redwood CA), The device used reversed iontophoresis for measuring interstitial glucose. It was noninvasive, worn as a wristwatch. However, it caused a lot of local irritation and was not a commercial success.

In 2004, Medtronic introduced wireless transmitting from sensor to receiver. It was possible to give alerts on high low glucose: that was significant improvement and became industry standard.

In 2006 Medtronic comes with Guardian REAL time CGM system with alerts on high and low glucose. By 2006 integrated pump and sensor was released.

Dexcom introduced its first real time sensor STS in 2006. The device needs calibration. The device needed calibration. The sensor lasted for 72 hours. It could be programmed to alert high and low values. The results could, however, not be used for clinical decisions- dvs that every result had to be checked by usual SBGM before change In insulin dosage.

In 2008 Abbott came with Free Style Navigator. The main advantage was longevity of the sensor – up to 5 days. But the equilibration (warm-up) time was up to 10 hours. The receiver had also a function as a glucometer: it was again necessary to check the result before changing the treatment.

In 2012 Dexcom G4 was available, now with a 7-day wear period. In 2015 it got FDA approval for use as aa CGM in patients ages 2–17. The same year A Dexcom G5 mobile platform was launched. That allowed for the CGM data to be transmitted to a compatible mobile device – users cell phone.

The last generation Dexcom G6 is a device that does not need calibration, lasts for 10 days and requires no confirmatory finger sticks. In 2018. Dexcom 6 became the first CGM to be approved by the FDA for integration in automated insulin dosing systems.

In 2016, Abbott introduced a new GCM device, Free Style Libre Pro Flash CGM, the first that does not require calibration. Initially, the system was indicated only for use by health care professionals and for use in the adult patients. The sensor could store the glucose data for up to 14 days. Glucose measurements were registered at 15 min intervals. But the system could not give real time data. The system was further upgraded to Free Style Libre 1 and 2, such that the patient can scan and get to know glucose levels. The system is allowed fro use in children older tah 4 years and in pregnant women.

In May 2016, Eversense introduced a CGM that included the only implantable glucose sensor with a 90 day lifespan. In 2017, Eversense XL was launched – with a lifespan of 180 days. To this day it is the CGM with the long- lasting glucose sensor available on the market.

Medtronic works in this period more on the integration of glucose sensor and insulin pump. In 2013 came MiniMed 530G sensor, the first pump with threshold suspends for hypoglycemia. Integration of CGM and insulin pump required also significant advantage in software, insulin algorithms and mobile technology. Today, integration of CGM with insulin infusion pumps includes both threshold and predictive low glucose suspend, as well as hybrid- and fully automated closed loop systems using either insulin alone or insulin and glucagon. The goal is to make an insulin pump that delivers insulin in accordance to sensed glucose, with truly little need for manual control of the device.

4. Glucose monitoring - what we do

Glucose monitoring is of proven clinical benefit in diabetes patients and it is the standard of diabetes medical care [10–12]. The possibility to move to capillary glucose measurement was significant for patient understanding of glucose variations, response to daily activities and effect of choices they make.

To summarize, we have several options that the health care provider and, more important, the patient can choose to follow with blood glucose levels.

- Glucometers-measure capillary blood glucose using fingerstick.
- Flash glucose monitors- measure interstitial fluid glucose by scanning of sensing device, intermittently.
- Continuous glucose monitors- a sensing device is continuously registering interstitial glucose levels. The data is sent to a device with real time check for viewing. Such devices can be integrated into insulin pumps.

We are aware of the classic glucose laboratory test is also in use and most used tests in modern laboratory medicine and are reference to accuracy, reproducibility and reliability of other methods.

It is also good to remember of some laboratory finesses that can be of significance if not observant in diagnosing diabetes.

Glucose can be measured in the whole blood, plasma or serum samples. Concentration of glucose is approximately 15% lower than in plasma or serum. Blood glucose cannot be decided accurately on postmortem specimens. Glucometers use capillary blood – also full blood that has a lower concentration of glucose than plasma. However, capillary blood has a higher concentration (up to 20%) than venous blood. Glucose concentration in samples that wait long for analysis are lower -because of glycolysis (and of course if not properly stored).

None of the devices is perfect and we must be aware of their limits. Not all the new devices are appropriate for all diabetes patients.

4.1 Blood glucose monitoring (BMG): self-blood glucose monitoring (SBGM)

Self-blood glucose monitoring is performed buy a glucometer. Capillary blood glucose is analyzed, using glucose oxidase or hexokinase methods.

It is the standard recommended glucose monitoring for most diabetes patients today.

Regular blood glucose monitoring (BGM) has been associated with improved glycemic control in T1D patients [10, 13]. Higher frequency of measurements is associated with lower HbA1c [14]. Evidence on the role of BGM in achieving optimal glucose control in patients with type 2 diabetes (especially the patients that are not using insulin) is limited [15–17]. It does, however, give BGM a significant new role in empowering the patient to live with diabetes.

4.2 Blood glucose monitoring: glucometers - glucose monitors

Glucose measuring devices analyze capillary blood glucose. The devices we use today give a reliable insight in glucose levels. Although great improvements since the first one that was in use, one must be aware that there are some analytical limitations of the devices (and not being sensitive enough in the low glucose range, is one of the most significant).

The accuracy of a glucometer is the parameter that is most important when deciding which ne to recommend and use. The question of accuracy and standardization is ongoing [18].

The highest standards are given by ISO and FDA. Standards vary depending on whether the device will be used by a professional or at home.

Marketed monitors in Europe must meet the following standard to be certified as accurate (dvs that the results can be used to make a therapeutic decision):

95% of the results must be within 15% of the reference method for blood glucose >100 mg/dl.

95% must be within 15 mg/dl for blood glucose <100 mg/dl.

For a glucometer to be certified by FDA, for use in diabetes patients, it is necessary that 95% of the results should be within 15% of the comparator method and 99% of results should be within +/−20% of the comparator across the entire claimed measuring range.

It is also necessary to perform adequately in the low glucose range: professional devices (used in the hospital) should achieve 95% of results within +/−12% of the comparator method for blood glucose levels >75 mg/dl (4,1 mmol/l) and within +/−12 mg/dl for levels under 75 mg/dl, they should achieve 98% of values within +/−15% of the comparator method for blood glucose levels >75 mg/dl and +/−15 mg/dl for levels <75 mg/dl across the entire claimed measuring range [19, 20].

BGM today is performed through a few simple steps. No matter how easy the steps may seem and no matter how accurate the system is, it is still possible to get a result that is inaccurate, because of the pre- or postanalytical errors. Some of the preanalytical errors are – poor skin preparation (having lotion or food rests on the skin, feks) or use of test strips that are incorrectly stored or expired. Postanalytical errors are mostly connected to registration of results, missing the values in the log, use of incorrect glucose units etc.

It is also estimated that only 7–13% of errors may occur during the analytical phase – if the patient is taking ascorbic acid or acetaminophen that will influence the results. Monitors that use glucose oxidase strips can give unreliable results when used bedside in patients that have oxygenation problems: low oxygen saturation will lead to false higher glycemia, while higher oxygen tensions in pat using oxygen may result I false ow glycemia. Monitors have also optimal range of working temperature. Test strips are most sensitive (again) to oxidation during improper or too long storage.

4.3 Blood glucose monitoring: the patient

One of the great changes in modern medicine, is moving from doctor- and medicine centered follow up of chronic diseases, towards patient empowered and disease mastering patient treatment. BGM is essential in such treatment concept in diabetes.

BGM is a standard of care and basic necessity for all patients with diabetes [21–23].

The significance of BGM is different in different groups of diabetes patients.

Also, the significance that BGM has for a patient is completely individual and are depending mostly on patient's motivation to integrate BGM in diabetes treatment plan.

4.3.1 Insulin treated diabetes type 1 patients

T1D patients on intensified insulin (multiple daily injections or CSII) treatment have, as previously mentioned, the greatest use of BGM based on their insulin regimen. It is recommended with monitoring in context of insulin dosage, postprandial, in mistaken hypoglycemia or hypoglycemia unawareness, after treating hypoglycemia, prior to exercise, prior to activity that requires normoglycemia (such as driving) or in the context of acute illness.

BGM with multiple daily monitoring in children and adolescents has special significance [24].

4.3.2 Gestational diabetes mellitus

Pregestational and gestational BGM is reduces HbA1c, but also the complications of diabetes pregnancies [25]. The recommendations ad requirements here are high:

Patients with known diabetes should plan pregnancy. In the pregestational period it is recommended that glucose monitoring be intense: pre breakfast, 2 h after all meals and at Bedtime.

Insulin dose should be titrated to achieve blood glucose.

4,0–5,8 mmol/l before breakfast.

>7,8 mmol/l post meal.

And 6-8 mmol/l at bedtime.

Once pregnancy is diagnosed intensive blood glucose monitoring is started, with the same glucose levels wanted): treatment is changed accordingly.

Pregnancy is surely the only glucose monitoring chapter with low tolerance for inconsistency.

How many times a day and in what order glucose should be monitored, is variable and has to be individualized also depending on what the goal is. In T1D patients on intensified insulin regime it is mainly insulin dosage that is the result of such monitoring. The intensity of BGM can also differ at different times, depending on patients specific needs at the time and patients goals at the time.

4.3.3 Diabetes type 2

Recommendations for patients that have T2D are a bit different: patients that use intensified insulin treatment should follow the recommendations as T1D patients.

Patients that use conventional treatment with basal insulin only can use BGM to titrate insulin dosage, but do, generally, not need intensified BGM.

Patients that do not use hypoglycemic drugs can have some help av. BGM, especially when adjusting diet, medications, level of activity or as a part of (introductory) diabetes treatment program.

Patients with prediabetes do not require self-blood glucose monitoring.

4.3.4 High accuracy

It is important to insist on devices with high accuracy (point of care requirements) glucose monitor in patients who [26].

1. Have a history of severe hypoglycemia or hypoglycemia unawareness

2. Are pregnant

3. Receive insulin therapy

4. Are otherwise at risk for hypoglycemia (feks use sulphonylureas).

5. Have occupations that enhance possible risks from hypoglycemia (fex driving or operating hazardous machinery).

6. Are using CGM device that uses calibration.

Its is necessary that all patients get god information and be educated to optimally use glucose meters, having in mind the major causes o eventually unreliable result.

4.4 Glucose monitoring: glucose monitors: what more is needed

Individual approach to every patient is important so that the recommendation on BGM (most of all structure of the measurements) leads to improved glucose control, but also improved feeling of diabetes control in patient self. It is important that the glucose value can be related to insulin dosage, meals, activity, illness, stress, new condition and that the patient/health care provider can get insight in glucose/diabetes dynamics, but also that they be able to conclude with a reasonable change. All the diabetes associations give some guidelines on number of necessary glucose measurements. But the number of required measurements must be in relation to patients needs. Gestational diabetes is maybe the only type of diabetes where the demand for BGM must be uncompromised.

But we must mention that it is often that the patient cannot follow with the requirements with BGM- it is not unusual to have patients that do not check blood glucose or do inconsequently. There are also patients who are not able to take appropriate self-management actions based on acquired data.

To motivate the patient for use of BGM can be a very complex and not always a successful job: although finger sticking can be the most intuitive hinder to multiple daily glucose measurements, it is not the main problem- BGM is a behavior and behavior is difficult to change without a structured plan and motivation [27–29].

BGM is the cornerstone of optimal diabetes management. It is important because it gives the patient direct insight into glycemia. It helps relate the symptoms to the number (hyper or hypoglycemia). It helps identifies hypoglycemia. The patterns and effects of different daily choices is obvious for the patient and health care provider. But, BGM gives us at discontinuous glycemic picture- there are periods of time that we do know nothing about blood glucose movements, periods with hypoglycemia or short postprandial hyperglycemia etc. That is an obstacle and hidden reason for patients' symptoms, daily function and obviously parameters of glucose control.

We hope that that is overcome today by the continuous glucose monitors.

5. Continuous glucose monitoring (CGM): significance

Continuous glucose monitor is, as previously mentioned, a device that can register interstitial glucose at short intervals. The results are sent o the receiver and are further used – stored or/and displayed for the patient. The device is a system of glucose sensor, transmitter, and receiver.

The use of CGM has brought the (patho) physiological glucose continuum in focus - there where it belongs. CGM today can provide real time glucose data 24 h/day, give alerts on imminent hypo- and hyperglycemia, show the rate of glucose level change. With help av. different algorithms the glucose levels can be used to show glucose change dynamics, periods with hypoglycemia TIR and so on.

From the first study where real time CGM was proved to reduce HbA1c and time spent in hypoglycemia [30], data is consistent. The use of CGM in patients on intensified insulin regime (with MII or insulin pumps) is associated with better HbA1, less time spent in hypoglycemia, less acute hypoglycemic events, and generally better satisfaction of patients. That covers many patient groups, also including diabetes type, gender, and age differences [30–35].

From the basic concept of CGM and first study it was clear that the CGM is most sensitive and useful in detecting and preventing hypoglycemia and time in hypoglycemic/near hypoglycemic range.

5.1 Continuous glucose monitoring - types

CGM devices can display real time data (CGM measures in short periods of time, presents real time data on the monitor, but also continuously stores data). Or CGM can continuously measure and store data, but gives the glucose level upon request, dvs when scanning the sensor.

CGM can be owned/used continuously by the patient intended for personal use. CGM can also be used by a professional- meaning that the CGM system is owned by the health care institution/provider: the patient gets the CGM over a period of time (7–14 days). The results may or may not be available for the patient at the time of use: the data are sent and stored at the doctor's office and analyzed retrospectively. Such short CGM periods can be useful for detecting daily patterns, vulnerable periods with hyper–/hypoglycemia.

The CGM measures glucose in the interstitial fluid. That means that the results we get are estimates- the numbers we get are somewhat "late" compared to the blood glucose. The greater rate of glucose level change in the circulation the greater "time lag", meaning also greater difference I the glucose level we get from CGM and BGM taken at the same time. That discrepancy is ameliorated by calibration or by integrated CGM algorithm. Not all the systems require calibration. But still, all the patients that have and use CGM, should have a blood glucose monitor available at all times- for eventual check on the CGM results (warm up periods, suspect hypoglycemia, lack of clinical correlation to hypo- alarm, fast change in glucose levels, lack of contact with the sensor etc..).

Some of the CGM (Dexcom G6- real time CGM and Free style Libre 2 - intermittently scanned CGM) can be integrated into insulin pumps. These CGM require no calibration.

5.2 Continuous glucose monitoring: some technicalities we have to consider

The sensitivity and accuracy of the CGMs is the subject of continuous improving. The mean absolute relative difference (MARD) is currently the most common metric used to assess the performance of CGM systems. MARD is the average of the absolute error between all CGM values and matched reference values. A small percentage indicates that the CGM readings are close to the reference glucose value, whereas a larger MARD percentage indicates greater discrepancies between the CGM and reference glucose values. MARD of <10% is considered sufficient to allow for therapeutic decision (insulin dose change).

CGM systems are sophisticated but it is not only the technical part that is responsible for eventual dysfunction. We are aware that the CGM is a foreign material that can cause allergic reactions. CGM must be inserter into the connective tissue. The actual connective tissue can be of different biological quality, variably circulated, the insertion is rarely the same etc. A sensor/glucose electrode can cause host response - irritation, immune reaction or inflammatory reaction or infection – the local process, no matter how complex, can change the sensitivity of the sensor. Sometimes it is only press on the sensor while sleeping that can provoke false alarm/ unreliable result.

Clinical situations that are associated with large body fluid shifts – dehydration, hypotension, hyperosmolality states, ketosis are not good ground for CGM function.

One must also be observant on substances that influence the glucose oxidase/ dehydrogenase systems.

The use of CGM should also be registered before major radiographic diagnostics.

CGM are expensive instruments and not evenly reimbursed. Optimal use of CGM requires a good educated health provider, a motivated and good educated patient and that of course implies a lot of time, not always available at the local doctor's office. Technical support, analyzing av. stored data (the need for compatible software, problems with personal safety when transmitting data etc. can also be a challenge [36, 37].

Patient motivation to understand the benefits and accept to wear CGM is also one of the critical factors for optimal use of CGM.

All this maybe explains that high quality CGMs are in use in about 50–75 pediatric endocrine practices and 35–50% in adult endocrine practices for individuals with T1DM [38].

5.3 CGM: The patient "who is capable of using devices safely"

The amount of data gathered on CGM was such that the ADA, in its Standards of care I 2020. states:

"when used properly, real time and intermittently scanned continuous glucose monitors in conjunction with insulin therapy are useful tools to lower A1c level and/or reduce hypoglycemia in adults with T1D who are not meeting glycemic targets, have hypoglycemia unawareness, and/or have episodes of hypoglycemia—and in conjunction to insulin therapy .. to lower A1C levels and/or reduce hypoglycemia in adults with type 2 diabetes who are not meeting glycemic targets" [39].

The 2022. Standards of Care recommend the use of real time continuous glucose monitoring (evidence level A) intermittently scanned continuous glucose monitoring (B) should be offered for diabetes management

- In adult patients with diabetes managed with multiple daily injections or CSII, who can use devices safely

- In youth with type 1 diabetes on multiple daily injections or CSII who are able to use the device safely 8 either alone or with a caregiver).

- In youth with diabetes type 2 on multiple daily injections or CSII who are capable of using the devices safely.

CGM, real time can be used for diabetes management in adults with diabetes on basal insulin who are capable on using the device safely.

Continuous glucose monitoring in adjunct to pre- and postprandial glucose monitoring can help achieve HBA1c targets in gestational diabetes.

Real time CGM should be used "as close to daily as possible" in patients using multiple daily injections or CSII for maximal benefit. Intermittent scanned CGMs should be scanned frequently, at least every 8 h.

The choice of CGM should be made based on patents "circumstances, desires and needs".

5.3.1 Gestational diabetes

The latest NICE guidelines do not differ significantly [40]. However, realtimeCGM should be offered to all pregnant women with type 1 diabetes, to help them meet pregnancy glucose targets an improve neonatal outcomes.

RT CGM should be considered for pregnant women that are on insulin therapy, not diabetes type 1, but have sever hypoglycemia (with or without impaired awareness of hypoglycemia). Or if they have unstable blood glucose levels. If CGM is already in use furthermore education and support should be provided by the antenatal/diabetes team [41].

As previously mentioned, the patient using CGM should always have a BGM available.

A large group of diabetes patients that have the need and desire for better glucose control can benefit for CGM. The patients who are, because of comorbidities, age etc., at increased risk for hypoglycemia or have poorly managed diabetes are candidates for real time or intermittent CGM, even periodically. But both the patient and the health care provider should be educated in use of CGM and both must be clear about the goals of CGM use. The patient (or, as nicely defined by the standards of care, caregiver) must be motivated to follow the message that CGM is sending and be able to respond properly. That would be the basis of GCM safety [42].

Of notice when considering safety is that the most advanced CGM are approved for use in children older than 2 years (Dexcom G6).

5.4 Continuous glucose monitoring: new glucose control parameters

Traditional methods of describing glucose control (HbA1c, BGM) are, now that we have a large amount of data from CGMs, not quite enough to fully describe glucose control and in most patients on intensified insulin regimes [43], not always enough to choose a proper therapeutic strategy.

5.4.1 Hypoglycemia

Hypoglycemia prevention and reduction of hypoglycemic episodes is one of the main advantages CGM can provide. But hypoglycemia in diabetes patient is sometimes difficult to define. The level of glucose, the rate of glucose level change and the duration of event is of significance. Originating form, the classic definition of hypoglycemia, CGMs register hypoglycemic events through two major intervals:

1. 3,9–3,0 (<70-54 mg/dl) mmol/l; That would be Level 1 hypoglycemia-hypoglycemia alert).

2. < 3,0mmoL/l (<54 mg/dl); that would be Level 2 hypoglycemia-clinically significant hypoglycemia, requiring immediate attention.

When defining hypoglycemia under CGM use, one should register the percentage of values below the named threshold (dvs percent of time with glycemia <3,9 mmol/l and percent of time spent under 3 mmol/, the later weighing heavier for the estimate); or the number of minutes/hours below the threshold. The number of such event should be reported. A significant event must last at least 15 minutes. Time spent in hypoglycemia should not exceed 1% for levels <3 mmol/l in adults with T1D, 4% for levels under 3,9 mmol/l.

In older adults time with hypoglycemia under 3,9 mmol/l should not exceed 1%.

5.4.2 Glucose variability

CGM has given us insight into different glucose patterns. Glycemic variability which reflects the amplitude frequency and duration of glucose fluctuation, is also a parameter that indicates the level of glucose control and is associated also with increased mortality in the ICU [44–46].

5.4.3 Time in range

Time in range is the time glucose measurements are in individual's target ("wanted") glucose range. TIR is giving some orientation about the time in eventual significant hyperglycemia or hypoglycemia. Such periods cannot be seen through HbA1c and discontinued capillary blood glucose measurements. Acceptable TIR for adults with type 1 diabetes is >70%, in older and high-risk patients >50%. Clinical benefits come with every 5% increment in TIR [47].

So, for complete insight in level of glucose control, optimal use av. data from CGM and right therapeutic decision we need to analyze far more parameters than HbA1c and the results of self-blood glucose monitoring, if any presented. Sufficient data is the data is 70–80% of possible CGM readings obtained for 2 weeks.

Here is a consensus on the parameters we should be aware of/analyze when analyzing CGM data.

(From: Battelino T, DanneT, Begenstal RM et al. Clinical targets for continuous glucose monitoring data interpretation: recommendations from the international Consensus on time in range: Diabetes care 2019; 42 [8]:1593–1603)

Standardized CGM metrics

1. Number of days CGM worn

2. Percentage of time CGM is active

3. Mean glucose

4. Estimated A1C

5. Glycemic variability (%CV or SD)

6. Time > 250 mg/dL (>13.9 mmol/L)

7. Time > 180 mg/dL (>10.0 mmol/L)

8. Time 70–180 mg/dL (3.9–10.0 mmol/L)

9. Time < 70 mg/dL (<3.9 mmol/L)

10. Time < 54 mg/dL (<3.0 mmol/L)

11. LBGI and HBGI (risk indices)

12. Episodes (hypoglycemia and hyperglycemia) 15 min

13. Area under the curve

14. Time blocks (24-h, day, night)

Use of Ambulatory Glucose Profile (AGP) for CGM report.

CV, coefficient of variation; LBGI, low blood glucose index; HBGI, high blood glucose index.

We believe that with such range of data to be considered, will the estimate of glucose control in diabetes patient is more adequate. If such analysis and, consequently estimate will be easier to get a therapeutic decision on, it is something that has to be seen. It is probably on the the next important mission, on GCMs integration with insulin pumps that the answer awaits.

6. Conclusion

It is difficult to imagine modern diabetes management without glucose monitoring. A number of devices help us get insight into diabetes of each and every patient and makes us intervene accordingly, for the short term and long-term benefit of the patient. It is only to expect that with constant improvement, glucose monitoring will continue to connect the patient, diabetes health care provider, but also the army of researchers, hardware and software developers, investors and people with great courage and ideas.

Although the advantages of glucose monitoring are beyond doubt, and are recommended clinical practice, there are still some obstacles to the broad and universal use of the different devices (lately the CGM devices). One of the main obstacles is certainly the cost of the devices. The reimbursement is variable. Availability is different in different parts of the world. The cost benefit is probably not considered from all levels of healthcare.

To optimally use glucose monitoring is not enough only to have the newest device. The educated health care provider (the choice and performances of devices, the analysis of data feks) and motivated and educated patient are also necessary to choose optimal way to use glucose monitoring. Enough time to educate, to obtain the data, to do the adequate analysis can be difficult to find in a busy practice and with an impatient patient.

Blood glucose monitoring is a daily task: although the devices and necessary routines are trending towards small, simple to use, easy to wear, easy to manipulate, easy to understand, "does it itself", it is necessary that the patient possesses a certain level of literacy and numeracy as well as knowledge on the method, so that the message on the monitor is understood and applied. Training in understanding and using the results to optimize glycemic management is necessary.

But, despite these impediments, the fact is that glucose monitoring has evolved and so has our understanding of diabetes and diabetes treatment. Technical advances are impressive.

There is a large diabetes population that expects to become free from multiple daily injections, bolus insulin dosage, fear for hypoglycemia and hypoglycemia. Integrating CGM in fully automated closed loop system, with insulin or combination with glucagon is maybe a way to open a new chapter in diabetes understanding and treatment. The high initial cost of implementing technology in everyday life of a diabetes patient and diabetes healthcare provider is still incomparable to the liberty such technology can give to the patient and to the satisfaction precisely tailored individualized successful treatment gives to both.

Author details

Anujka Selea Zivojinovic
Internal Medicine, Endocrinology, Medical Department, Aalesund Hospital, More og Romsdal HF, Norway

*Address all correspondence to: seleanujka@gmail.com

References

[1] Roberts JD, Caserio MC. The Structure and Properties of D-Glucose. Pasadena, CA: California Institute of Technology; 2021

[2] Clarke SF, Foster JR. A history of blood glucose meters and their role in self- monitoring of diabetes mellitus. British Journal of Biomedical Science. 2012;**69**(2):83-93

[3] Olczuk D, Priefer R. A history of continuous glucose monitors (CGMs) in self –monitoring of diabetes mellitus. Diabetes and Metabolic Syndrome-Clinical Research and Reviews. 2018;**12**:181-187

[4] Heller A, Ulstrup J. Detlev Muller's discovery of glucose oxidase in 1925. Analytical Chemistry. 2021;**93**(18):7148-7149

[5] Howell JO, Kaufman AD, Yeh HJ. Glucose test strips and electroanalytical chemistry in the undergraduate laboratory. Available from: https://www.basinc.com/assets/library/presentations/pdf/JOH-01.pdf

[6] Kohn J. A rapid method of estimating blood glucose ranges. Lancet. 1957;**273**(6986):119-121

[7] ADA Diabetes technology. Standards of care. Diabetes Care. 2021;**44**(Supplement-1):S85-S99

[8] UK Prospective Diabetes Study (UKPDS) Group. Intensive blood-glucose control with sulphonylureas or insulin compared with conventional treatment and risk of complications in patients with type 2 diabetes (UKPDS 33). Lancet. 1998;**352**:837-853

[9] Didyuk O, Econom N, Gaurdia A, et al. Continuous glucose monitoring devices: past present and future, focus on the history and technological innovation. Journal of Diabetes Science and Technology. 2021;**15**(3):676-683

[10] The Diabetes Control and Complications Trial Research Group. The Effect of Intensive Treatment of Diabetes on the Development and Progression of Long-Term Complications in Insulin-Dependent Diabetes Mellitus. New England Journal of Medicine. 1993;**329**:977-986

[11] Klein R. Hyperglycemia and microvascular and macrovascular disease in diabetes. Diabetes Care. Feb 1995;**18**(2):258-268

[12] American Diabetes Association. Consensus statement on self-monitoring of blood glucose. Diabetes Care. 1987;**10**(1):95-99

[13] Newton EJM, Ruta DA, et al. Frequency of blood glucose monitoring in relation to glycemic control: observational study with diabetes database. BMJ. 1999;**319**:83-86

[14] Miller KM, Beck RW, Bergenstal RM, et al. Evidence of a strong association between frequency of self -monitoring of blood glucose and HbA1c levels in T1D exchange clinic registry participants. Diabetes Care. 2013;**36**:209-214

[15] Farmer A, Wade A, Goyder E, et al. Impact of self-monitoring on blood glucose in the management of patients with non-insulin treated diabetes: open parallel group randomized trial. BMI. 2007;**336**:1174-1177

[16] Simon J, Gray A, Clarke P, Wade A, Neil A, Diabetes Glycemic Education and Monitoring Trial Group. Cost

effectiveness of self-monitoring of blood glucose in patients with noninsulin treated type 2 diabetes: economic evaluation of data from the DIGEM trial. BMJ. 2008;**336**:1177-1180

[17] Schwedes U, Siebold's M, Martes G. meal related structured self -monitoring of blood glucose: effect on diabetes control in nn-insulin treated type 2 diabetes patients. Diabetes Care. 2002;**25**:1928-1932

[18] US Food and Drug Administration. Self-Monitoring Blood Glucose Test Systems for Over the Counter Use: Guidance for the Industry and Food and Drug Administration Staff, US Food and Drug Administration. Available from: www.fda.god/regulatory-information/search-fda-guidance-documents/self-monitoring-blood-glucose-test-systems-over-counter-use-0

[19] US Food and Drug Administration. Blood Glucose Monitoring Test Systems for Prescription Point-of Care Use: Guidance by Industry and Food and Drug Administration Staff. US Food and Drug Administration. Available from: www.fdagod/regulatiry-information/search-fda-guidance-documents/blood-glucose-monitoring -test-systems-prescription-point-care -use

[20] Hagvik J. Glucose measurement: time for a gold standard. Journal of Diabetes Science and Technology. 2007;**1**(2):169-172

[21] Diabetes Technology. Standards of medical care in diabetes –2022. Diabetes Care. 2022;**45**(Suppl 1):S97-S112

[22] www.diabetes.ca/health-care -providers/clinical-practice-guidelines/chapter-9

[23] www.niddk.nih.god/health-information/diabets 7 overview/managing-diabetes/continuous-glucose-monitoring

[24] Ziegler R, Heidtmann B, Hilgard D, Hofer S, et al. DPV-Wiss-Initiative. frequency of SMBG correlates with HbA1c and acute complications in children and adolescents with type 1 diabetes. Pediatric Diabetes. 2011;**12**:11-17

[25] Siega-Riz AM, Viswanathan M, Moos MK, et al. A systematic review of outcomes of maternal weight gain according to the Institute of Medicine recommendations: birthweight, fetal growth, and postpartum weight retention. American Journal of Obstetrics & Gynecology. 2009;**201**(339):e1-339.e14

[26] Bailey TS, Grunberger G, Bode BW, et al. 2016 outpatient glucose monitoring consensus statement. Endocrine Practice. 2016;**22**:231-261

[27] Weinstock RS, Aleppo G, Bailey TS, Bergenstal RM, Fisher WA, Greenwood DA, et al. The Role of Blood glucose Monitoring in Diabetes Management. Arlington (VA): American Diabetes Association;

[28] Centers for Disease Control and Prevention. Diabetes Self-Management Education and Support (DSMES toolkit). Centers for Disease Control and Prevention; Available from: www.cdc.goc/diabetes/dsmes_toolkit/background/benefits.htlm

[29] Fisher WA, Kohut T, Stegner P, Schachner H. Understanding self-monitoring of blood glucose among individuals with type 1 and type 2 diabetes: an Information-Motivation-Behavioral Skills analysis. Diabetes Education. 2011;**37**:85-94

[30] Wv T, Beck RW, Bode BW, et al. Juvenile Diabetes Research Foundation Continuous Glucose Monitoring Study group. continuous glucose monitoring and intensive treatment of type 2 diabetes. New England Journal of Medicine. 2008;**359**:1464-1476

[31] Beck RW, Hirsch IB, Laffel L, et al. Juvenile Diabetes Research Foundation Continuous Glucose Monitoring Study Group: The effect of continuous glucose monitoring in well-controlled type 1 diabetes. Diabetes Care. 2009;**32**:1378-1383

[32] Vigersky RA. The benefits, limitations, and cost-effectiveness of advanced technologies in the management of patients with diabetes mellitus. Journal of Diabetes Science and Technology. 2015;**9**:320-330

[33] Klonoff DC, Buckingham B, Christiansen JS, et al. Endocrine Society: Continuous glucose monitoring: an Endocrine Society Clinical Practice Guideline. The Journal of Clinical Endocrinology and Metabolism. 2011;**96**:2968-2979

[34] Ehrhardt NM, Chellappa M, Walker MS, Fonda SJ, Vigersky RA. The effect of real-time continuous glucosemonitoring on glycemic control in patients with type 2 diabetes mellitus. Journal of Diabetes Science Technology. 2011;**5**:668-67532

[35] Baretlino T, Conget I, Olsen B, et al. SWITCH Study group te use and efficacy of continuous glucose monitoring in type 1 diabetes treated with insulin pump therapy: a randomized controlled trial. Diabetologia. 2012;**55**:3155-3162

[36] Beck RW, Riddelsworth T, Ruedy K, et al. Effects of continuous glucose monitoring on glycemic control in patients with type 1 diabets using insulin injections: the DIAMOND randomized clinical trial. JAMA. 2017;**317**:379-387

[37] Rodbard D. Continuous glucose monitoring: A review of success, challenges and opportunities. Diabetes Technology & Therapeutics. 2016;**18**(2):S2-3-S2-13

[38] Foster NC, Brown SA, LUmJW, Kovatchev BP. State of type 1 diabetes management and outcomes from the T1DExchange in 2016-2018. Diabetes Technology & Therapeutics. 2019;**21**:66-72

[39] American Diabetes Association. 7. Diabetes technology: standards of medical care in diabetes −2020. Diabetes Care. 2020;**43**(Suppl. 1):S77-S88

[40] www.nice.org. uk/guidance/ng17

[41] www.nice org.uk/guidance ng 3

[42] Miller EM. Using continuous glucose monitoring in clinical practice. Clinical Diabetes. 2020;**38**(5):429-438

[43] Danne T, Nimri R, Battelino T, et al. International consensus on use of continuous glucose monitoring. Diabetes Care. 2017;**40**(12):1631-1640

[44] Eslami S, Taherzadeh Z, Schultz MJ, Abu-Hanna A. Glucose variability measures and their effect on mortality: a systematic review. Intensive Care Medicine. 2011;**37**:583-593

[45] Battelino T, Danne T, Begenstal RM, et al. Clinical targets for continuous glucose monitoring data interpretation: recommendations from the International Consensus on time in range. Diabetes Care. 2019;**42**(8):1593-1603

[46] Vigersky RA, McMahon C. The relationship of hemoglobin A1C to time-in-range in patients with diabetes. Diabetes Technology & Therapeutics. 2019;**21**:81-85

[47] Roy W. Beck, Richard M. Bergenst MD et al. The Relationships Between Time in Range, Hyperglycemia Metrics, and HbA1c al, Journal of Diabetes Science and Technology 2019 13(4): 614-626

Chapter 5

Hypoglycemia Detection in Diabetes

James M. Richardson and Rimma Shaginian

Abstract

Hypoglycemia, once detected in a timely manner, is commonly treated by administration of glucose or glucagon in accordance with HCP advice, however, identifying the hypoglycemic event or need to treat is of initial paramount importance. The definition of hypoglycemia is provided, together with the implications of such an event on clinical and economic outcomes. The current accuracy standards are discussed and how they are applied to the low blood glucose range and current technologies.

Keywords: accuracy standards, blood glucose monitoring, continuous glucose monitoring, diabetes, hypoglycemia

1. Introduction

Diabetes is a lifelong, chronic disease characterized by episodes of hyperglycemia [1, 2]. Treatment of diabetes, in order to be effective, must lower glucose concentration to a euglycemic level, however, the key barrier to optimal glycemic control is hypoglycemia (low blood glucose levels) despite ongoing improvements in therapies and technology [3].

Hypoglycemia is one of the most impactful adverse events in diabetes and is a common problem for people with both type one (T1D) and type two (T2D) diabetes [4]. Too much insulin or, insulin-producing medications are commonly related to a hypoglycemic event, however other factors such as delayed, missed, or reduced meals other than what was planned, unanticipated strenuous exercise, alcohol consumption or interactions with other drugs are also known contributors. Additionally, individual patient factors such as older age, nutritional status, duration of diabetes, renal or hepatic disease, history of hypoglycemic episodes [5], and hypoglycemic unawareness may increase the risk of events [6].

2. The size of the problem

2.1 Hypoglycemia is the key problem in diabetes management

Despite recent advances in diabetes technology, hypoglycemia remains a key obstacle to achieving adequate glycemic control [3, 7, 8]. Even though the issue is well accepted, the size of the issue varies depending on how hypoglycemia is defined, measured, and reported. The incidence of hypoglycemia reported between randomized controlled trials vs. observational studies vs. patient-reported outcomes was found to differ by a factor of over 100 in one review [9].

2.2 Hypoglycemia is common problem for both T1D and T2D

The frequency of hypoglycemia varies from 42 to 91 events per patient year for adults with Type 1 diabetes (T1D) and from 20.3–44.4 events per patient year for adults with Type 2 diabetes (T2D) [10]. Severe hypoglycemia is not only a problem for insulin-treated patients but is also common among older adults with T2D across all levels of glycemic control. The risk tends to be higher in patients with either near-normal glycemia or very poor glycemic control [4]. Additionally, frequent episodes of mild hypoglycemia may compromise the hormonal counterregulatory response to produce adrenaline and subsequent autonomic warning symptoms such as trembling and sweating leading to hypo-unawareness increasing the risk of severe hypoglycemia further [6].

2.3 Clinical consequences of hypoglycemia are significant

With the general exception of diabetic ketoacidosis (DKA) and hyperosmolar hyperglycemic syndrome (HHS), the clinical consequences of prolonged hyperglycemia are long-term. These long-term risks were demonstrated in the Diabetes Control and Complications Trial (DCCT) [11] and the United Kingdom Prospective Diabetes Study (UKPDS) [12] for T1 and T2 diabetes respectively and are the result of neuropathy, retinopathy, and/or nephropathic complications.

The clinical consequences of severe hypoglycemia on the other hand can be immediately associated with the event and include acute cerebrovascular disease, myocardial infarction, neurocognitive dysfunction, and loss of vision [13]. If left untreated, severe hypoglycemia can result in significant morbidity and mortality [14, 15].

2.4 Economic consequences and human impact of hypoglycemia are significant

All levels of hypoglycemia are associated with significant indirect costs, not only on employers but also on individuals with diabetes [16]. A recent study showed a clear link between severe hypoglycemia and the costs of lost productivity, with the highest loss in productivity attributed to non-severe nocturnal hypoglycemic events [17]. Numerous studies have shown that hypoglycemia negatively impacts patients' ability to concentrate and participate in daily activities, thereby negatively impacting the quality of life (QoL) [17]. Even non-severe hypoglycemia, which occurs in 24–60% of patients with diabetes, can adversely affect QoL [18]. The greatest reductions in QoL are seen among those participants reporting a higher frequency of non-severe hypoglycemia [18]. As reported by Geelhoed-Duijvestijn et al., it takes an average of 50.4 min to return to normal functioning following a daytime non-severe hypoglycemic event, but negative feelings persisted for an average of 5.4 hours [19]. Following a nocturnal non-severe hypoglycemic event, functionality was diminished for an average of 80.5 min while negative feelings persisted for 12.2 hours [19].

Severe hypoglycemic episodes not only significantly affect the individual but are associated with long-term cost implications to the health system. One cohort study assessed the costs between a population requiring hospitalization due to severe hypoglycemia and a matched control. The results demonstrated that the group suffering from the severe hypoglycemic episode incurred an additional \$10,873 ($p < 0.001$) in direct and indirect costs vs. the control for that event year [20].

Hypoglycemia detection and management remain the cornerstone of modern diabetes management and it is important that patients and their healthcare providers (HCPs) understand the strengths and limitations of various blood glucose monitoring systems (BGMS) in order to select the most appropriate system that meets their individual needs [13].

3. Hypoglycemia definition and current threshold

3.1 Current classification of hypoglycemia

A joint position statement of the International Hypoglycemia Study Group of ADA and EASD has proposed three glucose severity levels when reporting hypoglycemia in clinical trials of glucose-lowering drugs for the treatment of diabetes (**Table 1**). The Group recommends that the frequency of detection of a glucose concentration < 3.0 mmol/l (<54 mg/dl), which it considers to be clinically significant biochemical hypoglycemia, should be included in clinical trial reports [21]. These levels are further aligned by the most recent version of the ADA's Standards of Medical Care in Diabetes 2022 (**Table 1**).

	ADA – Standards of Care 2022	**International Hypoglycaemia Study Group., 2017**
Level 1 < 70–54 mg/dL (3.9–3.0 mmol/L) with or without symptoms	Considered clinically important (independent of the severity of acute hypoglycemic symptoms)	This need not be reported routinely in clinical studies, although this would depend on the purpose of the study
Level 2 < 54 mg/dL (3.0 mmol/L) with or without symptoms	The threshold at which neuroglycopenic symptoms begin to occur and require immediate action to resolve the hypoglycemic event	Sufficiently low to indicate serious, clinically important hypoglycemia
Level 3 Severe hypoglycemia not defined by a specific glucose level	Defined as a severe event characterized by altered mental and/or physical functioning that requires assistance from another person for recovery	Severe cognitive impairment requiring external assistance for recovery

Table 1.
Levels of hypoglycemia proposed when reporting in clinical trials and as defined by the ADA.

4. Benefits and limitations of diabetes technologies assessing glucose levels

4.1 BGMS

4.1.1 Limitations of current ISO 2013 and FDA 2020 accuracy requirements for blood glucose monitoring systems in diabetes management

According to current ISO 15197:2013 accuracy requirements, ≥95% of BG results should be demonstrated to be within ±15% of the reference method for samples with BG concentrations ≥100 mg/dL, and ± 15 mg/dL when BG concentrations are <100 mg/dL. (International Organization for Standardization.)

The FDA guidance 2020 recommends that ≥95% of all BGMS results should be within ±15%, and ≥ 99% of all BGMS results should be within ±20% of the reference laboratory method across the entire claimed to measure range of the BGMS. (US Department of Health and Human Services [22]. Food and Drug Administration.)

These more stringent guidelines recognized the limitations of evaluating BG samples at the extreme ends of the measuring range, especially in the low range where very few samples are available [23]. Recognizing the clinical importance of the accuracy of BG measurements for hypo- and hyperglycemic blood samples, both European and US authorities have requested that accuracy data be reported separately for low, normal, and high BG ranges [23]. This issue is however complicated by system accuracy requirements being applied to measurement results from the whole glycemic range. If a BGMS shows 100% accurate results at BG concentrations ≥80 mg/dL (4.44 mmol/L) (80% of results, following ISO 15197:2013) [24], this results in 25% of the samples in the low-glucose range being allowed outside the accuracy limits (5% "results outside of accuracy limits" divided by 20% "results <80 mg/dL [4.44 mmol/L]") [23].

4.1.2 Difference of accuracy in hypoglycemic range of BGMS compliant with ISO 2013 standards and/or FDA 2020 guidelines

Despite the boundaries of ISO 2013 standards and/or FDA 2020 guidance, (International Organization for Standardization., US Department of Health and Human Services [22]. Food and Drug Administration) considerable differences exist in the performance of commercially available BGMS [25]. Such error patterns over the operating range of BGMS may lead to relevant differences in clinical and economic outcomes. These differences can potentially increase the risk of not detecting hypoglycemic events when they occur, and, therefore, inadequately identifying and treating them [25].

Thus, if a patient's true BG concentration is 60 mg/dL (3.33 mmol/L), acceptably accurate results range from 45 to 75 mg/dL (2.50 to 4.16 mmol/L) according to the ISO limits and from 51 to 69 mg/dL (2.83 to 3.83 mmol/L) according to FDA criteria. This can make it difficult for a patient to detect and manage their hypoglycemia. If a BGMS cannot reliably differentiate between 50, 60, and 70 mg/dL (2.77, 3.33, and 3.88 mmol/L), the utility of predefined hypoglycemia thresholds comes into question [23].

4.1.3 Evidence shows that the accuracy of different BGMS (compliant with ISO 2013) is not the same in the low-BG range

Multiple post-market studies of BGMS have failed to replicate the accuracy normally required to gain market approval by the regulatory authorities [26–30]. Many of these products remain on the market today.

Whilst it is not difficult to obtain BG samples in the normal range it is more of a challenge to obtain and subsequently assess the accuracy of devices outside of this range. It may be unethical and potentially dangerous to purposefully cause hypoglycemia in a patient simply for the purposes of testing device accuracy. The remaining choices to assess accuracy at this level is either to accept the smaller sample size, modify the sample prior to testing, or to create a statistical model. These concepts have further been explored in the low blood glucose range and evidence shows that the accuracy of different BGMS (that were approved under ISO 2013 standards) are not the same at these critical levels and some would appear non-compliant [29, 31]. Recently a methodology was developed to demonstrate the differences in accuracy in the low blood glucose range among several BGMSs as demonstrated in **Figure 1** [32–35]. The differences in accuracy between devices was clinically meaningful.

4.2 Continuous glucose monitoring technologies

Continuous glucose monitoring (CGM) devices have become more widespread over the past decade. They generally fall into two categories, real-time (rt-CGM) and intermittently scanned (is-CGM) devices. rt-CGM has shown positive improvements in improving HbA1c and reducing hypoglycemia in insulin users in RCTs [36–38] whereas is-CGM generally relies on observational data to support its use [39]. They predominantly differ from BGMS by measuring glucose concentration in the interstitial fluid, several times per hour, whereas BGMS measure blood (normally capillary) glucose once per test, up to around 10 times per day, depending on individual patient needs [1].

Unlike BGMS that have well-defined FDA and ISO accuracy criteria that must be met prior to obtaining marketing authorization, there remains no such standardized metrics for CGM accuracy requirements. In spite of this, it is commonplace for manufacturers to describe the accuracy of a CGM using Mean Absolute Relative Difference (MARD). This is calculated by averaging the absolute values of relative difference from the comparison method and does not account for positive or negative bias, i.e. all differences are made positive [40]. The MARD of some CGM systems has been reported to be in the 10–12% range whereas some BGMS has demonstrated to be below 5% [40].

One reason for the difference in MARD between some CGMs and BGMS could be attributed to measuring glucose in different compartments of the body. There is an inherent delay between glucose levels in each compartment with one study suggesting that to be between 6 and 10 minutes [41]. This makes it very difficult for a CGM to be as accurate, particularly at times of rapid glucose change. A further study demonstrated that MARD could change considerably throughout the day, approximately doubling between fasting periods and after food (8.0–16.3% and 9.1–16.3% depending on the device) [42]. This brings into question the value of such a metric if it can vary so much. **Table 2** provides some examples of when BGM is needed in CGM users.

Additionally, the detection of hypoglycemia by a CGM device is dependent on the duration of the hypoglycemic event. A recent study showed that two-thirds of all patients reported hypoglycemic events required minimum duration of 15 minutes in order to be by the CGM device [43].

A low ISF glucose reading below 3.9 mmol/L can prompt corrective actions that may be unnecessary if actual blood glucose, as measured by SMBG, is significantly higher. For instance, a user may develop hypoglycemia and take corrective action. Due to the time lag between blood glucose and ISF glucose, if the user continues to rely only on ISF glucose readings, there may be a lag in the rise of ISF over blood glucose, resulting in further and unnecessary treatment of hypoglycemia.

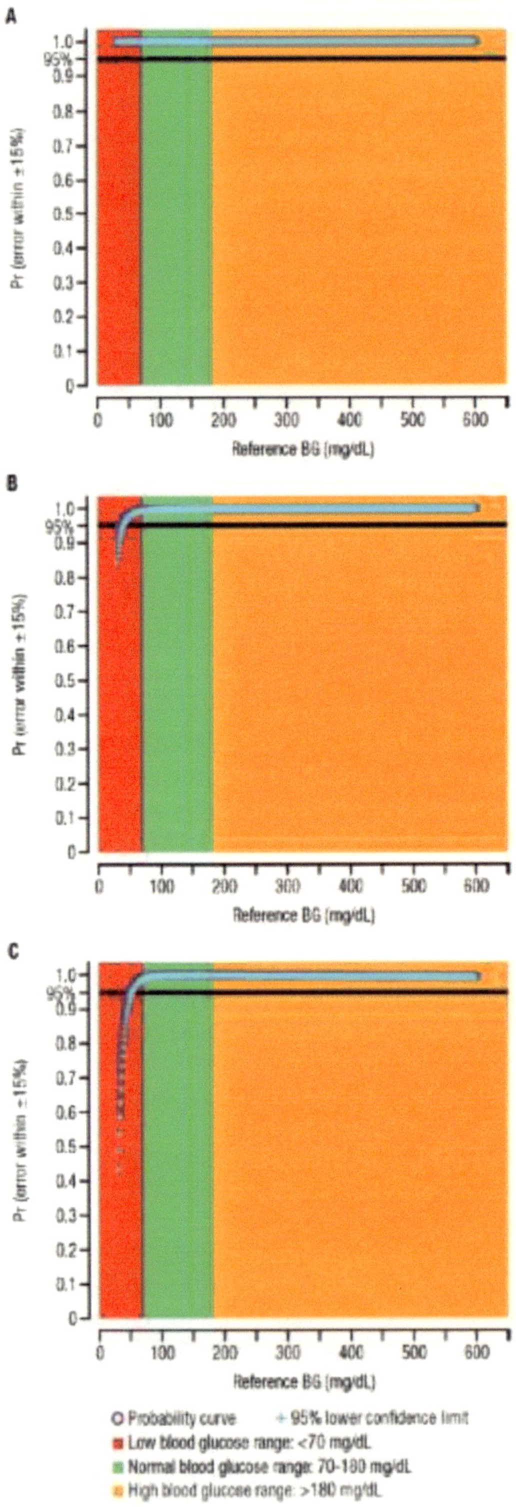

Figure 1.
Probability curves for real-world BGMSs (all meeting ISO 15197:2013 criteria) (adapted from [32]).

• During the first 24 h following sensor application when differences between blood glucose and ISF glucose are reportedly higher. This is hypothesized to be due to temporary local trauma at the site of application that affects ISF glucose concentration. The application of a new sensor 24 h before the old sensor "runs out" represents a potential solution to this issue.
• When a sensor glucose reading and trend arrow indicates a possible hypoglycemic episode or when symptoms suggest a hypoglycemic episode but the reader does not.
• Driving: To comply with both EU and UK legislation, the UK Driving and Vehicle Licensing Authority (DVLA) does not consider ISF glucose readings to be sufficient on their own and drivers must also monitor their blood glucose levels using a traditional blood glucose test. Naturally, this may change once there is more confidence in the accuracy of modern CGM and flash monitoring systems.
• Device-dependent interferences: When taking medications that have reported interference with ISF glucose values, for example, acetaminophen (paracetamol) or vitamin C (although this only applies to some ISF sensors).
ISF: interstitial fluid; CGM: continuous glucose monitoring; EU: European Union; and UK: United Kingdom.

Table 2.
Some examples for adjunct blood glucose testing in CGM users.

Similarly, experienced users may become less concerned with ISF low glucose readings than they would be with SMBG readings and take no immediate action. Each of these scenarios potentially creates unwanted risks [44].

The use of a CGM, particularly for the management of T1D, is preferred; however, all patients should learn how to use a BGMS for backup and monitoring if CGM is not available and/or desired [39]. This was further confirmed by the American Diabetes Association [1] which stated, "Every patient using a CGM must have a BGM." The reasoning for using a BGM when using a CGM includes whenever there is suspicion that the CGM is inaccurate, while waiting for warm-up, for calibration (some sensors) or if a warning message appears, and in any clinical setting where glucose levels are changing rapidly (>2 mg/dL/min), which could cause a discrepancy between CGM and BGM readings.

The definition of hypoglycemia is based on blood glucose readings, therefore the use of BGM in CGM users remains an essential part of their diabetes management.

5. Implications of hypoglycemia

5.1 Which diabetes patient needs the most accurate technology for hypoglycemia detection?

The American Association of Clinical Endocrinologists and American College of Endocrinology 2016 outpatient glucose monitoring consensus statement provided clinical situations and patients groups requiring the highest possible accuracy in glucose monitoring for detection of hypoglycemia [45]. These include those with a history of severe hypoglycemia; hypoglycemia unawareness; infants and children receiving insulin therapy; patients at risk for hypoglycemia, including patients receiving basal insulin or basal/bolus insulin therapy, patients with irregular schedules, skipped or small meals, vigorous exercise, travel between time zones, disrupted sleep schedules, shift work, and people with occupational risks that enhance possible risk from hypoglycemia (e.g., driving or operating hazardous machinery) [45].

Other patient groups include those receiving sulfonylurea or glinides [46], and people with diabetes with comorbidities such as hyperlipidemia or chronic renal disease who may also be taking multiple medications [47]. Age is also an important factor, as risk factors for hypoglycemia such as renal impairment, cardiovascular disease, and polypharmacy all increase with advancing age in adults with T2D [48–50].

The high accuracy in the low blood glucose range is also necessary for diabetes management during pregnancy, therefore CGM use in this patient population remains adjunctive use only [45, 51]. Blood glucose monitoring remains a cornerstone of glucose management during pregnancy [1].

6. Conclusions

In order to make correct therapy decisions, a correct glucose reading is essential [52]. In order to obtain a correct glucose reading, the correct device must be used. This selection spans both device types, i.e. CGM/BGM, and also specific device within the type. Accuracy variation within both system types is proven to be significant, therefore understanding the importance of education for HCP and patients to make an informed choice based on individual needs.

Acknowledgements

Medical writing was supported by Madano.

Conflict of interest

RS and JR are employees of Ascensia Diabetes Care Holdings AG.

Author details

James M. Richardson and Rimma Shaginian*
Ascensia Diabetes Care Holdings AG, Basel, Switzerland

*Address all correspondence to: rimma.shaginian@ascensia.com

References

[1] American Diabetes Association Professional Practice Comittee. 6. Glycemic Targets: Standards of Medical Care in Diabetes—2022. Diabetes Care. 2022;**45**(Supplement_1):S83-S96

[2] Schnell O, Hanefeld M, Monnier L. Self-monitoring of blood glucose: A prerequisite for diabetes management in outcome trials. Journal of Diabetes Science and Technology. 2014;**8**:609-614

[3] Cryer PE. Hypoglycemia: Still the limiting factor in the glycemic management of diabetes. Endocrine Practice. 2008;**14**:750-756

[4] Lipska KJ, Warton EM, Huang ES, Moffet HH, Inzucchi SE, Krumholz HM, et al. HbA1c and risk of severe hypoglycemia in type 2 diabetes: The Diabetes and aging study. Diabetes Care. 2013;**36**:3535-3542

[5] Anderson M, Powell J, Campbell KM, Taylor JR. Optimal management of type 2 diabetes in patients with increased risk of hypoglycemia. Diabetes Metab Syndr Obes. 2014;**2014**(7):85-94. Published 2014 Mar 6

[6] Clarke WL, Cox DJ, Gonder-Frederick L, Julian D, Kovatchev B, Young-Hyman D. Biopsychobehavioral model of risk of severe hypoglycemia. Self-Management Behaviors. Diabetes Care. 1999;**22**(4):580-584

[7] Cariou B, Fontaine P, Eschwege E, Lievre M, Gouet D, Huet D, et al. Frequency and predictors of confirmed hypoglycaemia in type 1 and insulin-treated type 2 diabetes mellitus patients in a real-life setting: Results from the dialog study. Diabetes & Metabolism. 2015;**41**:116-125

[8] Giorda CB, Ozzello A, Gentile S, Aglialoro A, Chiambretti A, Baccetti F, et al. Incidence and risk factors for severe and symptomatic hypoglycemia in type 1 diabetes. Results of the HYPOS-1 study. Acta Diabetologica. 2015;**52**:845-853

[9] Silbert R, Salcido-Montenegro A, Rodriguez-Gutierrez R, Katabi A, Mc Coy RG. Hypoglycemia among patients with type 2 Diabetes: Epidemiology, risk factors, and prevention strategies. Current Diabetes Reports. 2018;**18**(8):53

[10] Khunti K, Alsifri S, Aronson R, Cigrovski Berkovic M, Enters-Weijnen C, Forsen T, et al. Impact of hypoglycaemia on patient-reported outcomes from a global, 24-country study of 27,585 people with type 1 and insulin-treated type 2 diabetes. Diabetes Research and Clinical Practice. 2017;**130**:121-129

[11] Diabetes Control and Complications Trial Research Group, Nathan DM, Genuth S, et al. The effect of intensive treatment of diabetes on the development and progression of long-term complications in insulin-dependent diabetes mellitus. The New England Journal of Medicine. 1993;**329**(14):977-986

[12] UK Prospective Diabetes Study (UKPDS) Group. Intensive blood-glucose control with sulphonylureas or insulin compared with conventional treatment and risk of complications in patients with type 2 diabetes (UKPDS 33). [published correction appears in Lancet 1999 Aug 14;354(9178):602]. Lancet. 1998;**352**(9131):837-853

[13] Danne T, Nimri R, Battelino T, Bergenstal RM, Close KL, Devries JH, et al. International consensus on use of continuous glucose monitoring. Diabetes Care. 2017;**40**:1631-1640

[14] Griesdale DE, De Souza RJ, Van Dam RM, Heyland DK, Cook DJ, Malhotra A, et al. Intensive insulin therapy and mortality among critically ill patients: A meta-analysis including Nice-sugar study data. CMAJ. 2009;**180**:821-827

[15] Noh RM, Graveling AJ, Frier BM. Medically minimising the impact of hypoglycaemia in type 2 diabetes: A review. Expert Opinion on Pharmacotherapy. 2011;**12**:2161-2175

[16] Pawaskar M, Iglay K, Witt EA, Engel SS, Rajpathak S. Impact of the severity of hypoglycemia on health—Related quality of life, productivity, resource use, and costs among US patients with type 2 diabetes. Journal of Diabetes and its Complications. 2018;**32**:451-457

[17] Brod M, Christensen T, Thomsen TL, Bushnell DM. The impact of non-severe hypoglycemic events on work productivity and diabetes management. Value in Health. 2011;**14**:665-671

[18] Polonsky WH, Fisher L, Hessler D. The impact of non-severe hypoglycemia on quality of life in patients with type 2 diabetes. Journal of Diabetes and its Complications. 2018;**32**:373-378

[19] Geelhoed-Duijvestijn PH, Pedersen-Bjergaard U, Weitgasser R, Lahtela J, Jensen MM, Ostenson CG. Effects of patient-reported non-severe hypoglycemia on healthcare resource use, work-time loss, and wellbeing in insulin-treated patients with diabetes in seven European countries. Journal of Medical Economics. 2013;**16**:1453-1461

[20] Wong CKH, Tong T, Cheng GHL, et al. Direct medical costs in the preceding, event and subsequent years of a first severe hypoglycaemia episode requiring hospitalization: A population-based cohort study. Diabetes, Obesity & Metabolism. 2019;**21**(6):1330-1339

[21] International Hypoglycaemia Study Group. Glucose concentrations of less than 3.0 mmol/l (54 mg/dl) should be reported in clinical trials: A joint position statement of the American Diabetes Association and the European Association for the Study of Diabetes. Diabetologia. 2017;**60**:3-6

[22] US Department of Health and Human Services. Food and Drug Administration. Self-Monitoring Blood Glucose Test Systems for Over-the-Counter Use – Guidance for Industry and Food and Drug Administration Staff. 2020. Available from: https://www.fda.gov/media/87721/download [Accessed: January 2022]

[23] Heinemann L, Zijlstra E, Pleus S, Freckmann G. Performance of blood glucose meters in the low-glucose range: Current evaluations indicate that it is not sufficient from a clinical point of view. Diabetes Care. 2015;**38**:e139-e140

[24] International Organization for Standardization. In Vitro Diagnostic Test Systems—Requirements for Blood-Glucose Monitoring Systems for Self-Testing in Managing Diabetes Mellitus. ISO 15197. Geneva: International Organization for Standardization; 2013

[25] Budiman ES, Samant N, Resch A. Clinical implications and economic impact of accuracy differences among commercially available blood glucose monitoring systems. Journal of Diabetes Science and Technology. 2013;7:365-380

[26] Freckmann G, Baumstark A, Jendrike N, Zschornack E, Kocher S, Tshiananga J, et al. System accuracy evaluation of 27 blood glucose

monitoring systems according to DIN EN ISO 15197. Diabetes Technology & Therapeutics. 2010;**12**:221-231

[27] Freckmann G, Schmid C, Baumstark A, Pleus S, Link M, Haug C. System accuracy evaluation of 43 blood glucose monitoring systems for self-monitoring of blood glucose according to DIN EN ISO 15197. Journal of Diabetes Science and Technology. 2012;**6**:1060-1075

[28] Hasslacher C, Kulozik F, Platten I. Analytical performance of glucose monitoring systems at different blood glucose ranges and analysis of outliers in a clinical setting. Journal of Diabetes Science and Technology. 2014;**8**:466-472

[29] Klonoff DC. Postmarket surveillance of blood glucose monitor systems is needed for safety of subjects and accurate determination of effectiveness in clinical trials of Diabetes drugs and devices. Journal of Diabetes Science and Technology. 2019;**13**:419-423

[30] Pleus S, Baumstark A, Jendrike N, Mende J, Link M, Zschornack E, et al. System accuracy evaluation of 18 CE-marked current-generation blood glucose monitoring systems based on EN ISO 15197:2015. BMJ Open Diabetes Research & Care. 2020;**8**:e001067

[31] Freckmann G, Pleus S, Link M, Baumstark A, Schmid C, Hogel J, et al. Accuracy evaluation of four blood glucose monitoring Systems in Unaltered Blood Samples in the low glycemic range and blood samples in the concentration range defined by ISO 15197. Diabetes Technology & Therapeutics. 2015; **17**:625-634

[32] Pardo S, Shaginian RM, Simmons DA. Accuracy beyond ISO: Introducing a new method for distinguishing differences between blood glucose monitoring systems meeting ISO 15197:2013 accuracy requirements. Journal of Diabetes Science and Technology. 2018;**12**:650-656

[33] Richardson JM, Stuhr A, Pardo S, Shaginian RM. Challenges of hypoglycemia management using mobile applications. Oral presentation session 05. Diabetes Technology & Therapeutics. 2020:A-1-A-250

[34] Shaginian R, Richardson J, Pardo S, Stuhr A. Blood glucose monitoring systems' in the low blood glucose range and its clinical implications. Diabetes Technology & Therapeutics. No. S1A bstracts February 19-22, Madrid, Spain: The Official Journal of ATTD Advanced Technologies & Treatments for Diabetes Conference; 2020;**22**:A-1-A-250

[35] Stuhr A, Richardson JM, Pardo S, Shaginian RM. Accuracy of the contour®next one blood glucose monitoring system in the low blood glucose range using probability methodology. Diabetes Technology & Therapeutics. 2020;**22**:A-1-A-250. DOI: 10.1089/ dia.2020.2525.abstracts [Published Online: 18 Feb 2020]

[36] Bolinder J, Antuna R, Geelhoed-Duijvestin P, Kröger J, Weitgasser R. Novel glucose-sensing technology and hypoglycaemia in type 1 diabetes: A multicentre, non-masked, randomised controlled trial. Lancet. 2016;**388**(10057):2254-2263

[37] The Juvenile Diabetes Research Foundation Continuous Glucose Monitoring Study Group. Continuous glucose monitoring and intensive treatment of type 1 diabetes. The New England Journal of Medicine. 2008;**359**(14):1464-1476

[38] Van Beers CAJ, Devries JH, Kleijer SJ, Smits MM, Geelhoed-Duijvestijn PH, Kramer MHH. Continuous glucose monitoring for patients with type 1 diabetes and impaired awareness of hypoglycaemia (In control): A randomised, open-label, crossover trial. The Lancet Diabetes and Endocrinology. 2016;**4**(11):893-902

[39] Holt RIG, Devries JH, Hess-Fischl A, Hirsch IB, Kirkman MS, Klupa T, et al. The management of type 1 diabetes in adults. A consensus report by the American Diabetes Association (ADA) and the European Association for the Study of Diabetes (EASD). Diabetologia. 2021;**64**:2609-2652

[40] Freckmann G, Pleus S, Grady M, Setford S, Levy B. Measures of accuracy for continuous glucose monitoring and blood glucose monitoring devices. Journal of Diabetes Science and Technology. 2019;**13**(3):575-583

[41] Basu A, Dube S, Veettil S, Slama M, Kudva YC, Peyser T, et al. Time lag of glucose from intravascular to interstitial compartment in type 1 Diabetes. Journal of Diabetes Science and Technology. 2015;**9**(1):63-68

[42] Pleus S, Stuhr A, Link M, Haug C, Freckmann G. Variation of mean absolute relative differences of continuous glucose monitoring systems throughout the day. Journal of Diabetes Science and Technology. 20 Feb 2021;1932296821992373. DOI: 10.1177/1932296821992373. [Online ahead of print]

[43] Svensson CH, Henriksen MM, Thorsteinsson B, Pedersen-Bjergaard U. Continuous Glucose Monitoring (CGM) Readings during Patient-Reported Symptomatic. Hypoglycemia: Assessment of the Advanced Technologies and Treatments for Diabetes Consensus Definition of CGM-Recorded Hypoglycemia. Diabetes Technology & Therapeutics. Ahead of print; 2021. DOI: 10.1089/dia.2021.0216

[44] Ajjan RA, Cummings MH, Jennings P, Leelarathna L, Rayman G, Wilmot EG. Accuracy of flash glucose monitoring and continuous glucose monitoring technologies: Implications for clinical practice. Diabetes & Vascular Disease Research. 2018;**15**:175-184

[45] Bailey TS, Grunberger G, Bode BW, Handelsman Y, Hirsch IB, Jovanovic L, et al. American association of clinical endocrinologists and American college of endocrinology 2016 outpatient glucose monitoring consensus statement. Endocrine Practice. 2016;**22**:231-261

[46] Dunkley AJ, Fitzpatrick C, Gray LJ, Waheed G, Heller SR, Frier BM, et al. Incidence and severity of hypoglycaemia in type 2 diabetes by treatment regimen: A UK multisite 12-month prospective observational study. Diabetes, Obesity & Metabolism. 2019;**21**:1585-1595

[47] Alsahli M, Gerich JE. Hypoglycemia in patients with Diabetes and renal disease. Journal of Clinical Medicine. 2015;**4**:948-964

[48] Freeman J. Management of hypoglycemia in older adults with type 2 diabetes. Postgraduate Medicine. 2019;**131**:241-250

[49] Prinz N, Stingl J, Dapp A, Denkinger MD, Fasching P, Jehle PM, et al. High rate of hypoglycemia in 6770 type 2 diabetes patients with comorbid dementia: A multicenter cohort study on 215,932 patients from the German/Austrian diabetes registry. Diabetes Research and Clinical Practice. 2016;**112**:73-81

[50] Sinclair A, Dunning T, Rodriguez-Manas L. Diabetes in older

people: New insights and remaining challenges. The Lancet Diabetes and Endocrinology. 2015;**3**:275-285

[51] Immanuel J, Simmons D. A perspective on the accuracy of blood glucose meters during pregnancy. Diabetes Care. 2018;**41**:2053-2058

[52] Klonoff DC, Alexander Fleming G, Muchmore DB, Frier BM. Hypoglycemia evaluation and reporting in diabetes: Importance for the development of new therapies. Diabetes/Metabolism Research and Reviews. 2017;**33**:2883

Chapter 6

Treatment of Hypoglycemia

Yasin Simsek and Emre Urhan

Abstract

Hypoglycemia is an important condition that can be seen in everyone, more often in those with diabetes mellitus, and can sometimes be life-threatening. Hypoglycemia is a condition that can be prevented with simple precautions. It is a simple procedure that can be done mostly by ordinary people when the treatment is known. The most important step in the treatment is the education of those at risk of hypoglycemia and their relatives. The first step in treatment is to measure blood glucose, if possible. If blood sugar is below 70 mg/dl, hypoglycemia is diagnosed; if it is below 50 mg/dl, it is called severe hypoglycemia. The first approach in a conscious patient is to give the patient 15 mg of carbohydrate and measure the blood glucose again after 15 minutes. If the measured value is <70 mg/dl, the procedure should be repeated. If possible, glucagon should be administered to unconscious, out-of-hospital hypoglycemic patients until emergency help arrives. If glucagon is not available, glucose gel can be applied to the buccal mucosa. 50 ml of 50% glucose IV is administered to an unconscious hypoglycemic patient in the hospital. If the blood sugar does not rise above 70 mg/dl, the procedure is repeated.

Keywords: hypoglycemia, glucagon, glucose gel

1. Introduction

Hypoglycemia is generally considered to be a plasma blood glucose level of less than 4 mmol/L (70 mg/dL) in patients with diabetes mellitus. In general, the 'Whipple triad' (glycemia <50 mg/dL, symptoms suitable with low glycemia and these symptoms improve with a treatment that increases low glycemia) is sufficient for the diagnosis of hypoglycemia in persons with nondiabetics, although the plasma glucose level is above 50 mg/dL, most diabetic patients need treatment because of the symptoms of hypoglycemia [1].

2. Symptoms of acute hypoglycemia

It is divided into two main groups: adrenergic (neurogenic, autonomic) and neuroglycopenic [2]:

IntechOpen

2.1 Adrenergic signs and symptoms

It develops due to the activation of the autonomic nervous system and the adrenal medulla.

- Shaking.
- Cold sweats.
- Anxiety.
- Nausea.
- Palpitations.
- Numbness.

2.2 Neuroglycopenic signs and symptoms

It develops due to decreased glucose delivery to the cerebral cortex.

- Dizziness.
- Headache.
- İnability to concentrate.
- Difficulty speaking.
- Fatigue.
- Confusion.

3. Classification of hypoglycemia

Dividing symptomatic hypoglycemia into three according to the following clinical criteria is beneficial in terms of managing hypoglycemia;

3.1 Mild hypoglycemia

A condition in which the patient can detect and treat hypoglycemia ownself. Blood glucose is less than 70 mg/dL but is 54 mg/dL or higher.

Symptoms:

Sweating.
Shaking.
Nausea.
Extreme hunger.
Nervousness.
Dizziness.

3.2 Moderate hypoglycemia

It is the situation when the patient has to go to someone else's aid, but treatment is possible orally. Blood glucose is less than 54 mg/dL.

Symptoms:

Difficulty concentrating or speaking.
Confusion.
Weakness.
Vision changes.
Mood swings.

3.3 Severe hypoglycemia

When the patient is unconscious or unable to take oral glucose due to excessive disorientation and the treatment has to be administered parenterally as glucagon injection or intravenous glucose [3, 4].

Symptoms:

Confusion.
Dizziness.
Nausea or vomiting.
Shortness of breath.
Tremors or chills.
Extreme anxiety.
Irritability and changes in behavior.
Profuse sweating.
Pale, clammy skin.
Rapid heartbeat.
Extreme fatigue or sleepiness.
Loss of consciousness.
Seizures.

4. Treatment of hypoglycemia

4.1 Mild and moderate hypoglycemia

Mild hypoglycemic episodes can be prevented if a patient maintains a healthy diet and blood sugar levels are monitored regularly. For example, eating frequent small meals and having a few small snacks throughout the day will work in preventing hypoglycemia and keeping the patient's blood sugar under control. A good general rule is to eat six small meals each day, enough to meet your total daily carbohydrate needs. You should also drink plenty of water throughout the day. Treatment of mild hypoglycemia usually involves taking glucose tablets and/or foods containing simple sugars in case of hypoglycemia. However, this type of treatment is usually only necessary when you have no other choice. If patients continue to experience hypoglycemia despite following appropriate treatment and a healthy lifestyle, they should talk to their physician to revisal of their treatment [5].

Studies have shown that the glycemic response to oral glucose is transient, typically less than 2 hours. It was concluded that in the case of persistent or recurrent hypoglycemia, although oral glucose is effective, this is a temporary measure and may require a more substantial snack or meal followed by a meal. There is a "rules of 15" that recommends treating blood sugar <70 mg/dL by eating or drinking, a popular treatment strategy for mild hypoglycemia. 15 g carbs and repeat this treatment if symptoms persist after 15 minutes [6].

4.2 Severe hypoglycemia

Out of hospital: It is recommended that immediate administration of glucagon, if available, for the treatment of hypoglycemia in an unconscious person and in whom IV treatment is not possible. Administration of glucagon (subcutaneous, intramuscular, or nasal) will usually result in recovery of consciousness within about 15 minutes, although this may be followed by marked nausea and even vomiting. Therefore, the dose of glucagon should be followed by oral intake of concentrated carbohydrates just before the patient regains consciousness and nausea develops [7]. In the absence of glucagon, there are no conclusive data to guide the management of severe hypoglycaemia in patients with impaired consciousness who

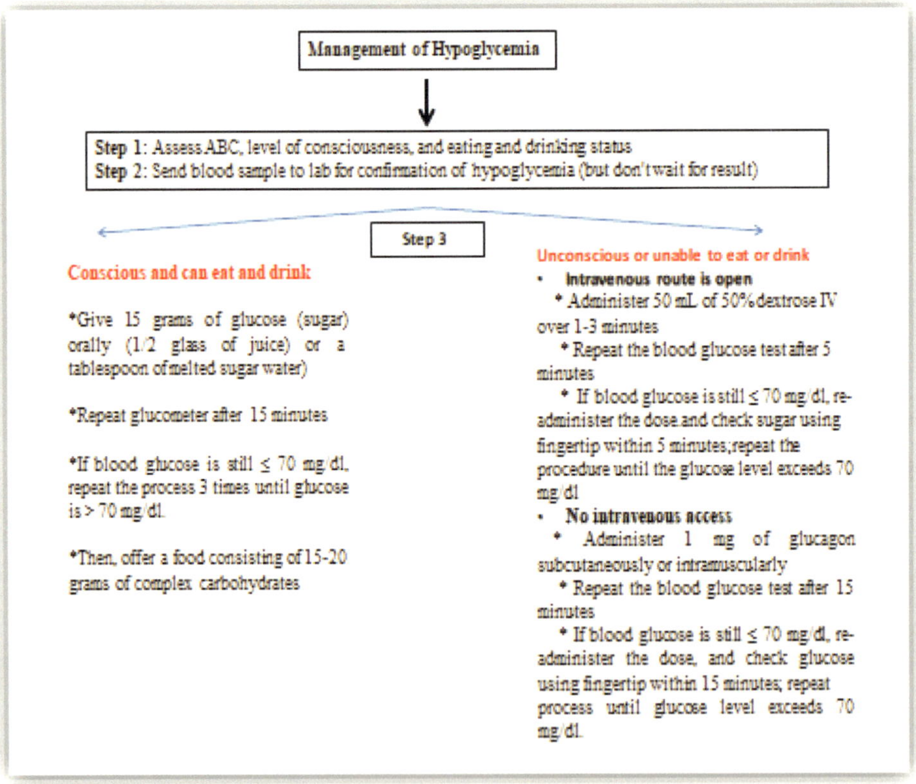

Figure 1.
Treatment of Hypoglycemia.

do not have immediate access to glucagon or intravenously (IV) dextrose (while emergency personnel are waiting). In a study on normoglycemic volunteers, buccal absorption of glucose was shown to be minimal. However, due to the lack of other options for such patients, some authors suggest that while awaiting emergency personnel, family members may apply a glucose gel (e.g., teeth and buccal mucosa) with the patient's head tilted slightly to the side [8]. If a glucose gel or pastry cream is not available There is some data showing that sprinkling table sugar under the tongue may be effective [9].

In hospital: Patients currently in the hospital can usually be treated quickly by administering 25 g of 50% glucose (dextrose) IV. Capillary blood glucose measurement must be repeated after 10 minutes. If it is still less than 70 mg/dL repeat IV glucose administration (**Figure 1**) [7].

5. Glucagon therapy

Glucagon exerts its hyperglycemic effects mainly by stimulating hepatic glycogenolysis. Unlike insulin, glucagon promotes catabolism and releases glucose [10]. Unlike other peptide hormones (e.g., insulin), glucagon does not show a clear dose-response relationship, suggesting that the glycemic response to glucagon is saturable. Increasing doses of glucagon do not result in a dose-dependent increase in glucose. Therefore, fixed doses are usually used. This situation has recently paved the way for the use of mini-doses of glucagon administered in doses of 100–150 μg instead of 1 mg to prevent or treat mild hypoglycemia [11].

5.1 Intranasal glucagon

Intranasal glucagon is a simple system that inserts the tip of the device into one nostril and empties the powder into the nostril. In a randomized trial comparing intranasal (3 mg) and intramuscular (1 mg) glucagon in patients with type 1 diabetes (T1DM) and hypoglycemia, hypoglycemia was successfully corrected in 98.7% and 100% of patients. The time taken for glucose values to rise above 70 mg/dL was 16 min for intranasal administration and 13 min for intramuscular administration [12].

5.2 Stable, liquid glucagon

Glucagon (or its glucagon analog) can be administered using a syringe kit as a pre-filled syringe containing a single-dose vial, all containing a fixed-dose, stable liquid glucagon preparation (dilution is not required) [13]. In studies in patients with type 1 diabetes, the improvement effects of hypoglycemia were similar in patients receiving 1 mg of stable liquid glucagon, 1 mg of reconstituted glucagon, or 0.6 mg of a glucagon receptor agonist (daciglucagon) [14].

5.3 Reconstituted glucagon

Glucagon lyophilized powder requires reconstitution just before use. It is administered subcutaneously or intramuscularly (1 mg). In an emergency, the dilution work may force the helpers into the environment [15].

6. Treatment of hypoglycemia in special cases

6.1 Strick glycemic control

In the treatment of diabetes, tight control is an important strategy in the prevention of microvascular complications. However, the morbidity and potential mortality of hypoglycemia are proven downsides of intensive glycemic management of diabetes [16]. There is strong evidence that tight glycemic control with insulin, sulfonylurea and glinide increases hypoglycemic morbidity and mortality in T1DM and type 2 diabetes (T2DM) [17, 18]. Therefore, alternative drugs with low hypoglycemic effect should be preferred if regulation can be achieved.

6.2 Lipohyperthyrophy at injection sites

Lipohyperthyrophy is an area of thickened subcutaneous fat tissue which is become due to the administering of continuous injection of insulin to the same area and incorrect rotation. When injecting insulin into the lipohypertrophic area, absorption is irregular, the rate of absorption is unpredictable and may cause glycemic fluctuations such as hypoglycemia [19]. Development of lipohypertrophy is preventable by changing the injection site (rotation) and not using insulin needles more than once [20].

6.3 Hypoglycaemia unawareness

Hypoglycemia unawareness (HU) refers to the occurrence of neuroglycopenia before the onset of warning symptoms in response to hypoglycemia. It is a condition that prevents strict diabetes regulation and reduces the quality of life, occurs in approximately 40% of people with T1DM and less frequently in T2DM [21]. Blood glucose monitoring, individualized goals and educational programs are important for the prevention and management of HU. Glycemic targets should be individualized, targeting less stringent regulation, especially for patients with long-standing diabetes, patients at high risk of HU and severe hypoglycemia, and/or patients with multiple comorbidities [22].

6.4 Severe hepatic dysfunctions

Hypoglycemia occurs when gluconeogenesis fails, especially in severe conditions such as liver failure where liver glycogen stores are reduced. The liver is one of the most important organs of glucose balance. Any disorders of its metabolism, structural integrity, or cellular functioning may impair the liver's ability to maintain normal glucose homeostasis. If such a disruption affects hepatic glucose output and gluconeogenesis, hypoglycemia may be occurred [23]. For patients with active liver disease, restrictive diets can often worsen protein-calorie malnutrition [24]. Most oral antidiabetic drugs are metabolized in the liver, and decreased glycogen stores are a risk factor for insulin-induced hypoglycemia, therefore strict monitoring of blood glucose levels should be performed during treatment in diabetic patients [25].

6.5 Impaired renal functions

Chronic kidney disease (CKD) can increase the risk of hypoglycemia. Decreased GFR is associated with decreased renal gluconeogenesis and clearance of insulin and other glucose-lowering drugs, and attenuation of the efficacy of regulatory mechanisms against hypoglycemia. Therefore, an individualized approach to diabetes management is essential, especially for patients with advanced CKD [26].

7. Prevention of hypoglycemia

Patient education, appropriate diet and exercise regimens, blood glucose monitoring, appropriate antidiabetic drug selection, and close clinical follow-up are necessary to prevent hypoglycemia [7].

7.1 Patient education

Patients and those around them should be educated about recognizing the symptoms of hypoglycemia and giving appropriate treatment for hypoglycemia as soon as possible. It is important to explain to patients the potential dangers of hypoglycemia and how it should be treated in patients treated with insulin, a sulfonylurea or glinide. Any documented hypoglycemia should be investigated with the patient to try to identify the causes, e.g., skipped meals/prolonged fasting, physical exertion, alcohol consumption, and injection of high insulin dose.

Diabetic patients at high risk of hypoglycemia are instructed to always carry glucagon with them. Family members and people around the patients with diabetes should be educated about the administration of glucagon to the patient; they also need to know where the glucagon is being held. There are subcutaneous, intramuscular injections, and intranasal forms of glucagon in the market.

7.2 Diet regulation

Dietary adjustment includes information about the amount of carbohydrates in meals and its effect on blood sugar concentration, and creating a personalized regular meal plan. The importance of administering insulin with the appropriate dose and timing regarding meals should be emphasized in patients receiving insulin therapy. Patients at risk of hypoglycemia should be advised to keep foods containing glucose or carbohydrates with them or in an accessible place. In some patients, especially those with T1DM or at high risk of nocturnal hypoglycemia, a bedtime snack may be recommended to prevent nocturnal hypoglycemia.

7.3 Recommendations on physical exercise

Physical exercise increases the risk of hypoglycemia by increasing glucose consumption. If necessary, early action can be taken to prevent hypoglycemia by measuring blood glucose before and after physical exercise. If there is a decrease in glucose level to the level of hypoglycemia, small meals should be eaten before physical exercise. Patients should be carried fast-acting carbohydrates with them during physical exercise. When planning physical exercise, it is important to adjust the insulin dose according to the exercise. Insulin doses should be reduced, more in heavy exercise and less in light exercise.

7.4 Medication adjustment

In patients receiving diabetes treatment, episodes of hypoglycemia may be associated with the treatment itself; therefore, it is important to use drugs with the low risk of hypoglycemia in such patients. Metformin, dipeptidyl peptidase-4 (DPP-4) inhibitors, glucagon-like peptide-1 (GLP-1) analogs, sodium-glucose cotransporter-2 (SGLT-2) inhibitors and pioglitazone are drugs with a low risk of hypoglycemia. In contrast, sulfonylureas and glinides are associated with a higher risk of hypoglycemia; Therefore, if treatment-related hypoglycemia occurs, it is recommended to consider reducing or discontinuing the dose of these drugs and switching to a different treatment [27].

With the transition to the use of long-acting basal insulin analogues (such as Detemir and Glargine U100), a significant reduction in nocturnal hypoglycemia attacks was achieved compared to Neutral Protamine Hagedorn (NPH) insulin [28]. The new ultra-long basal insulins Glargine U300 and Degludec have recently led to a significant additional reduction in the rate of nocturnal hypoglycemia [29]. The use of short-acting insulin analogs has resulted in a significant reduction in the rates of severe hypoglycemia compared to conventional human insulin [30].

Author details

Yasin Simsek[1]* and Emre Urhan[2]

1 Endocrinology and Metabolism Department, Acibadem Hospital, Kayseri, Turkey

2 Endocrinology and Metabolism Department, Erciyes University, Kayseri, Turkey

*Address all correspondence to: yasinsimsek79@gmail.com

References

[1] Cryer PE, Axelrod L, Grossman AB, et al. Endocrine Society. Evaluation and management of adult hypoglycemic disorders: An Endocrine Society Clinical Practice Guideline. The Journal of Clinical Endocrinology and Metabolism. 2009;**94**(3):709-728

[2] Slama G, Traynard PY, Desplanque N, et al. The search for an optimized treatment of hypoglycemia. Carbohydrates in tablets, solution, or gel for the correction of insulin reactions. Archives of Internal Medicine. 1990;**150**(3):589-593

[3] ISPAD International Society for Paediatric and Adolescent Diabetes Consensus Guidelines 2000; Classification of Hypoglycaemia. Available from: http://www.diabetesguidelines.com/health/dwk/pro/guidelines/ispad/13_03.asp [Accessed: October 18, 2012]

[4] Sua YJ, Liao CJ. Hypoglycemia in emergency department. Journal of Acute Disease. 2015;**4**(1):59-62

[5] Delahanty LM, Halford BN. The role of diet behaviors in achieving improved glycemic control in intensively treated patients in the Diabetes Control and Complications Trial. Diabetes Care. 1993;**16**(11):1453-14588

[6] Wiethop BV, Cryer PE. Alanine and terbutaline in treatment of hypoglycemia in IDDM. Diabetes Care. 1993;**16**(8):1131-11366

[7] Diabetes Canada Clinical Practice Guidelines Expert Committee, Yale JF, Paty B, Senior PA. Hypoglycemia. Canadian Journal of Diabetes. 2018;**42**(1):104-108

[8] Gunning RR, Garber AJ. Bioactivity of instant glucose. Failure of absorption through oral mucosa. Journal of the American Medical Association. 1978;**240**(15):1611-1612

[9] Barennes H, Valea I, Nagot N, et al. Sublingual sugar administration as an alternative to intravenous dextrose administration to correct hypoglycemia among children in the tropics. Pediatrics. 2005;**116**(5):648-653

[10] Kulina GR, Rayfield EJ. The role of glucagon in the pathophysıology and management of diabetes. Endocrine Practice. 2016;**22**(5):612-621

[11] Blauw H, Wendell DVJH, et al. PCDIAB consortium. Pharmacokinetics and pharmacodynamics of various glucagon dosages at different blood glucose levels. Diabetes, Obesity & Metabolism. 2016;**18**(1):34-39

[12] Rickels MR, Ruedy KJ, Foster NC, et al. Intranasal glucagon for treatment of insulin-induced hypoglycemia in adults with type 1 diabetes: A randomized crossover noninferiority study. Diabetes Care. 2016;**39**(2):264-270

[13] Valentine V, Newswanger B, Prestrelski S, et al. Human factors usability and validation studies of a glucagon autoinjector in a simulated severe hypoglycemia rescue situation. Diabetes Technology & Therapeutics. 2019;**21**(9):522-530

[14] Beato-Vibora PI, Arroyo-Diez FJ. New uses and formulations of glucagon for hypoglycemia. Drugs Context. 2019;**8**:212599

[15] Isaacs D, Clements J, Turco N, Hartman R. Glucagon: Its evolving role

in the management of hypoglycemia. Pharmacotherapy. 2021;**41**(7):623-633

[16] Hemmingsen B, Lund SS, Gluud C, et al. Intensive glycaemic control for patients with type 2 diabetes: Systematic review with meta-analysis and trial sequential analysis of randomised clinical trials. BMJ. 2011;**343**:d6898

[17] ORIGIN Trial Investigators, Mellbin LG, Ryden L, Riddle MC, et al. Does hypoglycemia increase the risk of cardiovascular events? A report from the ORIGIN trial. European Heart Journal. 2013;**34**(40):3137-3144

[18] McCoy RG, Van Houten HK, Ziegenfuss JY, et al. Increased mortality of patients with diabetes reporting severe hypoglycemia. Diabetes Care. 2012;**35**(9):1897-1901

[19] Omar MA, El-Kafoury AA, El-Araby RI. Lipohypertrophy in children and adolescents with type 1 diabetes and the associated factors. BMC Research Notes. 2011;**12**(4):290

[20] Cho NH, Shaw JE, Karuranga S, et al. IDF diabetes atlas: Global estimates of diabetes prevalence for 2017 and projections for 2045. Diabetes Research and Clinical Practice. 2018;**138**:271-281

[21] Vignesh JP, Mohan V. Hypoglycaemia unawareness. The Journal of the Association of Physicians of India. 2004;**52**:727-732

[22] Martin-Timon I, Del Cazzo-Gomez FJ. Mechanisms of unawareness of hypoglycemia and implications in diabetic patients. World Journal of Diabetes. 2015;**6**(7):912-926

[23] Norris ML, Harrison ME, Isserlin L, et al. Gastrointestinal complications associated with anorexia nervosa: A systematic review. The International Journal of Eating Disorders. 2016;**49**(3):216-237

[24] Tolman KG, Fonseca V, Dalpiaz A, Tan MH. Spectrum of liver disease in type 2 diabetes and management of patients with diabetes and liver disease. Diabetes Care. 2007;**30**(3):734-743

[25] Garcia-Champion D, Gonzalez-GonzalezJA,Lavalle-GonzalezFJ, et al. The treatment of diabetes mellitus of patients with chronic liver disease. Annals of Hepatology. 2015;**14**(6):780-788

[26] Ahmad I, Zelnick LR, Batacchi Z, et al. Hypoglycemia in people with type 2 diabetes and CKD. Clinical Journal of the American Society of Nephrology. 2019;**14**(6):844-853

[27] American Diabetes Association. 9. Pharmacologic approaches to glycemic treatment: Standards of medical care in diabetes-2021. Diabetes Care. 2021;**44**(1):111-124

[28] Monami M, Marchionni N, Mannucci E. Long-acting insulin analogues versus NPH human insulin in type 2 diabetes: A meta-analysis. Diabetes Research and Clinical Practice. 2008;**81**(2):184-189

[29] Gerber AJ, King AB, Del Prato S, et al. NN1250-3582 (BEGIN BB T2D) Trial Investigators. Insulin degludec, an ultra-longacting basal insulin, versus insulin glargine in basal-bolus treatment with mealtime insulin aspart in type 2 diabetes (BEGIN Basal-Bolus Type 2): A phase 3, randomised, open-label, treat-to-target non-inferiority trial. Lancet. 2012;**379**(9825):1498-1507

[30] Pedersen-Bjergaard U, Kristensen PL, et al. Effect of insulin analogues on risk

of severe hypoglycaemia in patients with type 1 diabetes prone to recurrent severe hypoglycaemia (HypoAna trial): A prospective, randomised, open-label, blinded-endpoint crossover trial. The Lancet Diabetes and Endocrinology. 2014;**2**(7):553-561